Prelude to Hospice

Critical Issues in Health and Medicine

Edited by Rima D. Apple, University of Wisconsin–Madison,
and Janet Golden, Rutgers University, Camden

Growing criticism of the U.S. health care system is coming from consumers, politicians, the media, activists, and health care professionals. Critical Issues in Health and Medicine is a collection of books that explores these contemporary dilemmas from a variety of perspectives, among them political, legal, historical, sociological, and comparative, and with attention to crucial dimensions such as race, gender, ethnicity, sexuality, and culture.

For a list of titles in the series, see the last page of the book.

Prelude to Hospice

~

Florence Wald, Dying People, and their Families

EMILY K. ABEL

Rutgers University Press

New Brunswick, Camden, and Newark, New Jersey, and London

First paperback edition 2020
ISBN 978-0-8135-9392-0

Library of Congress Cataloging-in-Publication Data

Names: Abel, Emily K., author.
Title: Prelude to hospice : Florence Wald, dying people, and their families /
Emily K. Abel.
Description: New Brunswick, New Jersey : Rutgers University Press, [2018] | Series:
Critical issues in health and medicine | Includes bibliographical references and index.
Identifiers: LCCN 2017053034 | ISBN 9780813593913 (hardback : alk. paper) |
ISBN 9780813593937 (e-pub) | ISBN 9780813593951 (Web PDF)
Subjects: | MESH: Wald, Florence. | Hospice Care—history |
History, 20th Century | Hospices—history | United States
Classification: LCC RA999.H66 | NLM WB 310 | DDC 362.17/56—dc23
LC record available at https://lccn.loc.gov/2017053034

A British Cataloging-in-Publication record for this
book is available from the British Library.

∞ The paper used in this publication meets the requirements of the
American National Standard for Information Sciences—Permanence of Paper
for Printed Library Materials, ANSI Z39.48-1992.

www.rutgersuniversitypress.org

Manufactured in the United States of America

Contents

Contents

Prelude to Hospice

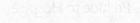

Introduction

Hospices have played a critical role in transforming ideas about death and dying. They emerged in the late 1960s, a time of growing concern about the use of aggressive, high-tech treatments at the end of life. The hospice movement views death as a natural event and seeks to enable people approaching mortality to live as fully and painlessly as possible. Its founder was Florence Schorske Wald, the former dean of the Yale University School of Nursing, who was committed to advancing social justice and applying the psychoanalytic thought that had begun to transform her profession.

Wald's remarkable study of terminally ill people and their families occupied a central place in her campaign to establish the first U.S. hospice. Because the study never was published, it has received little attention. Fortunately, however, Yale University's Sterling Memorial Library has preserved the notes of the researchers' interactions with patients and relatives as well as their discussions of the cases with other health professionals and investigators. Although some records are missing, the extant ninety files provide a wealth of information that sheds new light on hospice history.[1]

In a 1986 article titled "The Hospice Movement: Institutionalizing Innovation," I noted that the early U.S. hospice movement expressed a number of ideals that distinguished it from the established health care system. As hospices grew in number and popularity, however, they were gradually incorporated into the mainstream and lost their uniqueness.[2] Six years later, "The

Routinization of Hospice," an article by sociologists Nicky James and David Field, made a similar argument about the United Kingdom. The first UK hospices were established outside the National Health Service to encourage innovation, but routinization and bureaucratization soon blunted their distinctiveness.[3]

Reviewing those two papers, historian David Clark recently asked whether they "betray a somewhat romantic nostalgia on the part of historians and sociologists removed from the daily realities of delivering hospice services" or "grasp the nettle of an issue likely to prove problematic . . . if ignored."[4] The records this book analyzes suggest that both characterizations are valid. Because most early U.S. hospices tried to adhere to Wald's principles, her detailed notes of her interactions with patients, families, and other health professionals may be as close as we can come to understanding the day-to-day work of those programs. The records indicate that hospices have departed from their initial ideals not only because they merged with the mainstream but also because those ideals were always difficult to fulfill. But the records also suggest that hospices have long provided a compassionate alternative to high-tech hospital care that is still desperately needed.

Wald launched "The Nurses Study of Dying Patients and Their Families" (later renamed the "Interdisciplinary Study of Dying Patients and Their Families") soon after returning from London in 1968. There she had visited St. Christopher's in the Field, the first modern hospice, founded by social worker, nurse, and doctor Cicely Saunders. Wald envisioned the study as the first step in founding a similar facility in the United States. In 1974, Hospice Inc. (later the Connecticut Hospice) opened in New Haven, Connecticut, providing home care services to people with a limited life expectancy, a primary caregiver at home, and a cancer diagnosis. Six years later, the hospice established an inpatient facility in Branford.

Following Saunders, Wald asserted that the suffering of dying people had social and emotional components as well as physical ones. As a result, she assembled an interdisciplinary team to help her conduct the research. The initial members included another nurse, a pediatrician, an oncologist, and a Methodist minister. Doctors at Yale New Haven Hospital (YNHH) referred patients to the study; eligibility criteria included a life expectancy of approximately three months and residence in the greater New Haven area. Both patients and their families had to agree to be studied; in return, they received special care. Seven months after the research began, the investigators decided to restrict participants to breast cancer patients on the oncologist's roster. A $25,000 grant from the U.S. Public Health Service enabled Wald to devote half of her time to the study. As principal investigator, she not only directed the research but also nursed the patients she studied. She usually spent twelve hours a week on patient care but increased her time when death seemed close. By spring 1971, she had cared for twenty-two patients and their families.

Both Wald and the other nurse involved in the study kept handwritten logs of all their interactions with patients and their family members. An administrative assistant later typed those reports. The entire research team discussed the cases at monthly meetings with other health professionals, which were recorded and transcribed. Beginning in fall 1970, Wald met regularly with Donna Diers, a professor at the Yale School of Nursing and an expert on research methodology; their meetings also were recorded and transcribed. In addition to the logs and transcriptions, the records contain other miscellaneous items, including letters from patients, relatives, and doctors; medical records; newspaper clippings; and speeches and articles by the researchers and other experts.

Although several sociological accounts of medical care for dying people had appeared recently, Wald stressed the uniqueness of her study. She was interested in family members as well as patients, followed both groups over time, and interviewed patients not only in acute care hospitals but also in chronic care facilities and at home. In fund-raising appeals, Wald enunciated various goals. The primary one was to understand the wants and needs of dying people and their families. Because patients' most pressing concern was symptom relief, Saunders had devoted considerable energy to developing a new method of pain control. As a nurse rather than a doctor, Wald could not follow Saunders's example in that regard. She worked closely with both a doctor and a pharmacist with a special interest in pain medication, but she concentrated on other issues.

Wald was a complex figure. Dedicated to improving terminal care and inspiring others to join her mission, she deserves much of the credit for launching the U.S. hospice movement. Like other great visionaries, however, she could sometimes be intolerant of people who disagreed with her. The study gave her the first opportunity to apply her methods about how to treat people confronting death. Influenced by the Freudian psychology that was popular at the time, she framed the needs of the people she studied in therapeutic terms. She asserted that both patients and their families must express their feelings openly, share them with each other, and resolve all tensions among them. When people followed her prescription, the dying process could be a growth experience and death serene.

Adopting the role of participant observer, Wald interpreted her duties as a nurse extremely broadly. In addition to providing physical care, she did housework, ran errands, helped children with homework and drove them to and from school, and provided psychological advice; in at least one case, she introduced study participants to members of her own family. As a result, she often established profound relationships with the people she cared for. Interviewed in 2017, her son Joel recalled her deep attachment to one man. Because he lived in the next town, she visited frequently. "I remember my mother dropping everything whenever she received a call from the man's wife or one of his children, often driving off into the night to spend hours at their house,"[5] Joel recounted. But some of her actions transgressed conventional boundaries and violated psychoanalytic teachings about transference and countertransference. Intensely involved in the personal lives of people she studied, she occasionally became entangled in family conflicts and tensions.

In addition to helping understand the prelude to the hospice movement, the detailed records analyzed in this book enable us to glimpse the various ways patients and their kin experienced and responded to the approach of death in the late 1960s and early 1970s. The book also provides a unique window on end-of-life care during that period. The researchers carefully analyzed the interactions between physicians and patients just when that relationship was beginning to undergo transformation. A growing number of patients began to feel emboldened to challenge doctors' authority, demanding information about diagnosis and treatment and participation in decision-making. Numerous scholars point to two studies to demonstrate a dramatic shift in authority relations. In 1961, Donald Oken concluded that 90 percent of physicians did not tell their patients they had cancer.[6] Using Oken's questionnaire, Dennis H. Novack reported in 1979 that 97 percent of physicians did inform patients they had cancer, a stunning reversal.[7] Wald's records suggest that the contrast between those studies may be less significant than scholars suggest. Both Oken and Novack based their findings on what doctors claimed to do. Scrutinizing the practices of physicians, Wald found that even those who proclaimed the importance of truth-telling employed various strategies to conceal bad news. Although doctors' changing attitudes toward medical secrecy have received considerable attention, there is little information about patients' responses. Wald's records indicate that some patients accepted the misinformation they received, but others began to distrust the doctors who hid what they knew to be the truth.

Death moved into hospitals more slowly than birth, but half of all people died there by 1960, and many patients who died elsewhere enrolled in those facilities during the last year of life.[8] In addition, growing numbers of critically ill patients spent their last days in intensive care units (ICUs). Six years after North Carolina Memorial Hospital in Chapel Hill established the first ICU in 1953, a survey found 238 units in short-term, private nonprofit hospitals. By 1965, the number had grown to 1,040.[9] And in both ICUs and regular hospital rooms, patients at the end of life increasingly received complex technological care. Wald's study confirmed the findings of recent sociological accounts that hospital doctors often tried to sustain life long after there was any hope for recovery. She had wanted to teach hospital personnel about her new model of care. The negative response she received reinforced her belief that the hospice she planned should be completely divorced from the established health care system.

Wald was especially shocked when she suspected that the therapies dying people received were not in their best interests. As a major academic medical center, YNHH had a large research enterprise. A rapidly proliferating literature describes the way investigators treated human subjects, but we have little insight into the subjects' responses to participation in medical studies. Wald and her colleagues extensively recorded the experiences of a wealthy white woman who underwent an experimental procedure and then entered the hospital research ward for follow-up studies. Another large body of literature demonstrates that clinical trials in the United States historically relied disproportionately on vulnerable populations, including poor people, people of color, prisoners, and inmates of institutions for mentally retarded children.[10] But some people with high social status have served as research subjects, especially if they were believed to be close to death. The experiences of the socially prominent participants in clinical studies are important for two reasons: their sense of entitlement made them unusually sensitive to abuse, and others were more likely to listen to their complaints and take them seriously. Although the patient Wald studied gave consent, she later regretted having done so. Several observers substantiated her charge that the treatment violated her dignity and exposed her to harm. It seems likely that many members of the vulnerable populations who participated in clinical trials received care that was even less respectful and therapeutic.

This book also examines one of the first attempts to test Elisabeth Kübler-Ross's theory. Eleven months after Wald inaugurated the study, Kübler-Ross's book *On Death and Dying* appeared. Based on observations of dying hospital patients, she argued that people close to death passed through five emotional stages—denial, anger, bargaining, depression, and finally acceptance. Her book rapidly became a best seller, and many people still use it to understand grief. Because the theory supported many of Wald's ideas about the dying process, she too embraced it. But when she and her colleagues tried to fit their data into Kübler-Ross's paradigm, they reluctantly concluded that the model imperfectly described the psychological responses of most people confronting mortality. The researchers were especially troubled by Kübler-Ross's assumption that everyone must achieve acceptance, a notion that remains widespread.

Although Wald had intended to publish an academic study, she felt overwhelmed by the wealth of data and eventually abandoned the effort. But she often presented her material informally. On such occasions, she departed sharply from her findings to make the case for a new type of medical facility. For example, she offered generalizations that had little basis in her data. In addition, she carefully selected the cases she discussed and then embellished them. Like many others seeking to found new institutions, she believed she could garner support by demonstrating that what her facility offered would be superior in every respect to what currently existed. As a result, she generated inflated expectations about what a hospice could accomplish.

Perhaps Wald also needed to convince herself that she knew how best to facilitate a good death. Historian Drew Gilpin Faust analyzed the condolence letters penned by Civil War soldiers to bereaved families of dead comrades. Letter after letter sought to demonstrate that the fallen had achieved the ideal of a good death not because the writers ignored contrary evidence but because they needed to "maintain the comforting assumptions about death and its meaning with which they had begun the war. In the face of the profound upheaval and chaos that civil war brought to their society and to their own individual lives, Americans North and South held tenaciously to deeply rooted beliefs that would enable them to make sense out of a slaughter that was almost unbearable."[11] In far less terrible circumstances, Wald desperately wanted to believe that her model of care could foster a peaceful death despite the misery she continually observed. Even today, many obituaries assert that the patient died peacefully, surrounded by family, although the reality may have been very different. Despite the recent efforts to increase awareness and acceptance of death, we remain hesitant to acknowledge the suffering it often entails.

Chapter 1 examines the background of Wald's study. Like many historians, I begin with Saunders's visit to the United States in 1963, when she lectured widely about her research on pain control and her vision for the hospice she planned to establish in London. But U.S. hospices were not simply a British import. I focus less on the content of Saunders's message than on the reasons her American audiences so enthusiastically embraced it. The chapter discusses the early history of Wald and her most prominent colleagues, criticisms of hospital care for dying people that had emerged in the late 1950s, and contemporaneous movements for social change both at Yale University and in the surrounding community.

Believing that teamwork was a central component of the hospice mission, Wald hoped to eliminate status differentials between herself and doctors. That hope was quickly dashed. Chapter 2 explores her relationship with the physician she found most sympathetic to her cause, who became a key member of her research team. He gave some credence to her concerns about research on human subjects but ignored many of her other comments and suggestions, especially about truth-telling.

The following two chapters present case studies that introduce recurrent themes. Both indicate that applying Wald's ideals of terminal care was far more difficult than she initially imagined. Chapter 3 discusses an elderly Italian immigrant man with a large family. He had been ill for several months before entering the study, and his doctors expected him to die soon. Although Wald frequently referred to a family as "the unit of care," this one was torn by dissension. Wald allied herself first with one side and then the other. The major conflict concerned how aggressively the patient should be treated while he continued to outlive the doctors' predictions. Unable to communicate easily with the many family members who spoke little English, the researchers viewed them as stereotypical Italian immigrants.

Chapter 4 tells the story of a forty-year-old widow whom Wald met in the YNHH breast cancer clinic. Sharing both life circumstances and interests with her, Wald was able to forge a close relationship and offer emotional as well as medical and practical support. Family tensions focused on plans for the woman's three adolescent daughters after she no longer could care for them. An even more serious clash erupted between Wald and the patient's sister, leading Wald to withdraw much earlier than she had planned.

Chapter 5 examines the major themes that emerged from Wald's study, including her biases and those of other researchers, their assessments of the advantages and disadvantages of various sites of death, and debates about the meaning of acceptance. The chapter then explores the uses Wald made of her findings. Ironically, her scrupulous record-keeping enables us to perceive the enormous gap between the experiences of many terminally ill people and their kin and the idealized image she presented. The chapter juxtaposes descriptions of events in her daily log with the accounts she gave in articles, speeches, and informal talks.

As a participant observer, Wald tried to apply her principles of care while studying patients and their kin. As the research proceeded, she continued to proclaim the benefits of those principles while concealing the many obstacles she encountered. Although we lack detailed accounts of the day-to-day activities of early hospices, it is likely that they confronted similar impediments. The conclusion demonstrates that the histories of those hospices similarly ignored the complexities of the work of tending dying people and their families. In addition, I argue that despite their inability to realize all their goals, those programs provided a model of humane care that is threatened not only by integration into the mainstream but even more by the growing dominance of for-profit entities.

1

Setting the Stage

Saunders "just opened the door to me," Wald recalled. Saunders "solved the problem that both the faculty and the students were having in the hospital, seeing patients, particularly cancer patients, being treated with curative treatment, and where it was very obviously not curing the disease, but the suffering was so great. . . . They couldn't get the doctors to tell them what was . . . the outlook for them, or to consider a variety of ways of treating the situation."[1] Saunders traced her interest in end-of-life care to her work with a Jewish immigrant from the Warsaw ghetto who was dying in a London hospital. She then gained additional experience caring for terminally ill people at two other London facilities: St. Luke's Hospital and St. Joseph's Hospice. By 1963 when Saunders traveled throughout the United States, she had developed a new method of pain control and begun planning St. Christopher's, the hospice she established in London four years later. In talk after talk, she chastised doctors who concluded there was "nothing more to be done" for patients desperately needing pain relief and spiritual and emotional solace. At Yale she received a standing ovation. Although Wald, then dean of the nursing school, was not in the audience, she heard about it from a colleague and soon established a close relationship with Saunders. Throughout the rest of her life, Wald referred to Saunders as her primary mentor.[2]

Born in New York City in 1917, Wald noted that she learned to value social justice as a child. Her father was a banker and her mother a secretary. Although neither attended college, she described them as "very vigorously self-educated." They also "were very liberal in their thinking." Her father subscribed to *The Nation*, and both parents registered as Socialists and championed Norman Thomas. Her mother volunteered at a health care clinic serving poor people.[3] Religion, however, had no place in the family. Although her father was Christian by background and her mother Jewish, Wald stated that both were "free thinkers, and really never depended on religion as their spiritual resource throughout their life, even through death." Wald's father complained that the churches took too much money from people.[4] He appears to have had a special antipathy toward Catholicism, the religion of half the participants in Wald's study. Her father led the family on Sunday morning walks and "as we passed the Catholic church when the congregants were saying Hail Marys, he would shake his walking cane at the church and shout 'Papist pap for the masses.'"[5] Throughout her life, Wald railed against the harm caused by organized religion.[6] According to her daughter Shari Vogler, however, Wald's husband was born into an orthodox Jewish family. When they married, they agreed to bring up their children as Jewish. They belonged to a conservative synagogue and celebrated the High Holidays and Passover.[7]

Wald graduated from Mount Holyoke in 1938 and the Yale School of Nursing in 1941. Her first job was at Henry Street Nurses Settlement, established by Lillian Wald in New York's Lower East Side. (Although Florence liked people to associate her with Lillian Wald, they were not related.) By the time Lillian Wald retired in 1933, the nursing service had cared for 100,000 patients, many of whom were immigrant and poor.[8] Florence Wald was disappointed to find it had changed dramatically when she arrived in 1942. As she told an interviewer, "it was not really helping the impoverished or the disadvantaged" but was "just nursing. It didn't have its social component."[9] She left in 1944 to enter the U.S. Army Signal Corps and then worked as a research assistant in two medical facilities. In 1953, she joined the nursing staff at New York's Babies Hospital. Founded in 1887 by two physicians who

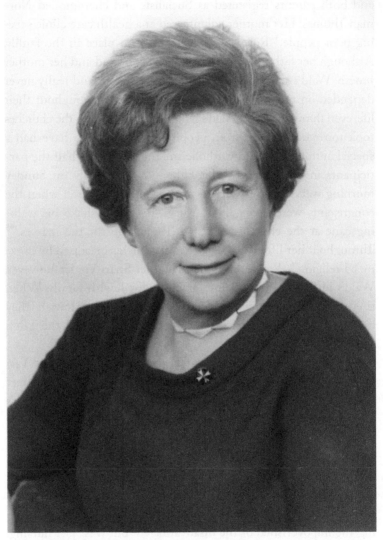

FIG. 1. Florence Schorske Wald
(Credit: Yale University, Harvey Cushing/John Hay Whitney Medical Library)

were sisters, Babies Hospital served children younger than three. During the 1920s, it was affiliated with Columbia-Presbyterian Hospital.[10]

At Babies Hospital, Wald began to join an interest in psychiatry to her long-standing commitment to social justice. In that period, psychiatry increasingly meant Freudian psychoanalysis. As a past president of the American Psychiatric Association noted, "By 1960, almost every major psychiatry position in the country was occupied by a psychoanalyst," and "the psychoanalytic movement had assumed the trappings of a religion."[11] Wald was introduced to the field by reading Anna Freud's writings about the impact on children of separation from their parents. Deciding to pursue her new interest, Wald enrolled in an MS program in Mental Health Nursing at Yale in 1955. There she met Ida Orlando, one of three professors who influenced Wald by integrating mental health theories into nursing. Wald wrote that Orlando "urged students and colleagues to encourage patients to express their thoughts and feelings about the illness and proposed treatment," a practice that later became central to Wald's writing and work.[12]

In 1956, Wald joined the faculty of Rutgers University School of Nursing to work under Hildegard E. Peplau, who had adapted Henry Stack Sullivan's theory of interpersonal relations to nursing practice in her landmark 1952 book *Interpersonal Relations in Nursing: A Conceptual Frame of Reference for Psychodynamic Nursing*. She urged nurses to develop close personal relationships with patients, empathize with their feelings of anxiety, grief, and anger, and help them complete unfinished psychological tasks. To perform that work well, Peplau encouraged nurses to act as participant observers, carefully studying the patients they cared for. Peplau, like Orlando, advocated a new direction for a field dominated by rigid rules and routines. "Nurses dealt with patients only when they had something in their hands—a thermometer, a lunch tray, medications, or a bedpan," Peplau's biographer explained. "Talking to patients in any substantial way was discouraged."[13] Peplau noted that her theory also helped nurses demarcate a unique sphere of competence. Since the early 1900s, physicians had become increasingly distant from their patients. Medical schools encouraged students to protect themselves against patient suffering. The growth of specialization and the expansion of medical technology further separated physicians and patients. Peplau argued that rather than passively executing doctors' orders, nurses must draw on their particular expertise, countering the medical depersonalization patients had begun to criticize. She had an especially profound impact on Wald.[14] In future chapters, I will show how Wald incorporated many of Peplau's ideas into her own, defining herself as a participant observer, arguing that patients must complete unfinished business, and emphasizing the therapeutic potential of her relationships with them.

In 1957, Wald returned to Yale School of Nursing, then considered the premier nursing school in the country, as a professor of psychiatric nursing.[15] The following year, she married Henry Wald, an engineer whose wife had died suddenly, leaving him with two young children. Florence thus added parenting to her other obligations. By the time of her study on dying people, Joel was a student at Yale and Shari a junior in high school. Henry offered Florence unqualified support and encouragement. He listened to her daily accounts of relationships with the patients and families in her study and occasionally interacted with them himself. He also embraced her goal of establishing the hospice, providing professional as well as emotional assistance. Soon after she began her study of dying people, he closed his engineering practice to enroll in the Columbia University School of Architecture, specializing in health care facilities. His 1971 MA thesis, "A Hospice for Terminally Ill Patients," was instrumental in planning the inpatient unit of the Connecticut Hospice.[16]

Wald was appointed dean of the school of nursing in 1959. Donna Diers, a faculty member in the school, noted that Wald was eager to promote nursing research and made contact with August B. Hollingshead, chair of the sociology department.[17] It is likely Wald was especially interested in his *Social Class and Mental Illness: A Community Study* (1958), written with psychiatrist Frederick C. Redlich. Wald also saw early drafts of *Sickness and Society*

(1968), which was based on a study Hollingshead had conducted at Yale New Haven Hospital (YNHH) with pediatrician Raymond Duff, who later served as a consultant in Wald's own study. Diers's admiration for Wald did not extend to her management style: "She had her hands in everything. It made us crazy. She was given to walking into our offices (often when we had just been whingeing about the Dean) to follow up on a prior conversation, making us flush with guilt. It was eerie. It wasn't really micromanagement but it felt intrusive."[18] We can assume that Wald brought that style to her interactions not only with other researchers and health professionals but also with the people she studied.

One of Wald's closest nursing school colleagues was Virginia Henderson, another major critic of what she called "regimentalized patient care" and "the concept of nursing merely ancillary to medicine," as well as a proponent of developing nurse-patient relationships.[19] Wald undoubtedly appreciated the attention Henderson gave to care for dying people. "In talking about nursing," Henderson wrote in 1966, "we tend to stress promotion of health and prevention and cure of disease. We rarely speak of the inevitable end of life and what the nurse might do to help a person reduce its physical discomforts—to face death courageously, with dignity, and even bring to it an awesome beauty."[20] Immediately after attending Saunders's 1963 lecture at Yale, Henderson rushed to tell Wald what she had heard. Although we cannot know exactly what Saunders said, Henderson's description three years later suggests that Saunders greatly exaggerated her ability to provide a good death: "She shows one photograph after another of a person eating a meal, sitting in a chair in the ward or on the terrace, knitting, or occupied with a game, and she says, not without pride, that he died three days later, or 'He died peacefully the next day.'"[21] There was, apparently, no mention of anyone suffering uncontrollable pain, gasping for breath, or hallucinating. We will see that one of the many ways Wald followed Saunders's example was by romanticizing deaths that occurred under hospice care.

After hearing Henderson's account, Wald arranged a special luncheon for Saunders and then began a correspondence and invited her to speak at the school in 1965. In 1966, Saunders returned to Yale for six weeks, and the following year Wald took a sabbatical at St. Christopher's Hospice, now operating in London. Soon after her return, she resigned her position as dean to devote herself to establishing the first U.S. hospice. The first step was to study dying patients and their families.

Saunders had coined the phrase "total pain" to emphasize that the suffering of dying people had spiritual and emotional components as well as physical ones.[22] As her student, Wald assembled an interdisciplinary team to assist her research. In addition to herself, the primary members were Ira S. Goldenberg, an oncologist surgeon and professor at Yale Medical School; Morris A. Wessel, a pediatrician; Edward Dobihal, chaplain at YNHH and a faculty member of the Yale Religious Department; and Katherine Klaus, another nurse. Wald later noted that the group added "at times" Frederick Auman, the minister of Trinity Evangelical Lutheran Church, and Robert Canny, a Catholic priest.[23] Given her emphasis on psychological growth, it may seem strange that Wald did not invite any psychiatrists to join her. Two members of the group, however, shared her interest in psychiatry.

After receiving a divinity degree from Drew Theological Seminary in 1952, Dobihal served as pastor at a Methodist church in Jersey City and then as a chaplain at St. Elizabeths Hospital, a government psychiatric hospital in Washington, DC. While there Dobihal studied at the Washington School of Psychiatry and conducted research for a doctoral dissertation on the psychological and religious dimensions of bereavement. In 1964, he left St. Elizabeths for Yale and the following year received his PhD in human relations from Drew University.[24]

Wessel later described the monthly meetings of the research team "as a giant oasis in an institution where technological progress and piecemeal professional care minimized the possibility of helping patients live fully and with dignity to the end."[25] Born in 1917, he received his BA from Johns Hopkins University in 1939 and MD from Yale Medical School in 1943. After serving in the Army, he became a pediatric fellow at the Mayo Clinic in Rochester,

Minneapolis, and then a research fellow at Yale Medical School. By 1968 he had been in private practice in New Haven for eighteen years and become one of the city's most popular pediatricians.[26]

Although Wessel had no formal training in psychoanalysis, he was greatly influenced by two doctors who did. At the Mayo Clinic, he worked under Dr. Benjamin Spock, who had attended the New York Psychoanalytic Institute and later relied on Freud's theories in his best-selling books on baby and child care.[27] (In 1993, Spock praised Wessel as one of the first pediatricians to focus on children's emotional development.[28] Five years later, Wessel described Spock as "a vitally important mentor" throughout his career.[29]) As a research fellow at Yale, he provided assistance to Edith Jackson's famous study on "rooming in," the practice of letting newborns remain with their mothers rather than automatically placing them in central nurseries. A psychoanalyst as well as a pediatrician, Jackson had undergone a six-year analysis with Freud and studied at the Vienna Psychoanalytic Institute.[30] Wessel attributed his interest in end-of-life care to his father's death when Wessel was eleven months old, the terminally ill children he met in his practice, and the concerns of the many parents who had endured traumatic experiences with mortality in childhood. In addition, he noted the similarity between Jackson and Saunders. Both taught him "to understand and respect and admire the way human beings meet the exigencies of life at the momentous occasions of becoming parents or at the moment of death."[31]

Goldenberg explained the absence of psychiatrists on the research team by noting that he and most other members were qualified to deal with any emotional problems that arose. After serving in the Army during World War II, he had received a BA from the University of Michigan and an MD from Boston University. Between 1952 and 1957, he worked first as an intern and then a resident in surgery at Yale University School of Medicine. He joined the school's faculty in 1957, becoming a clinical professor of surgery in 1968.[32]

Goldenberg's career success at Yale could not have come easily. The surgeon and award-winning author Sherwin B. Nuland recalled that when he entered Yale School of Medicine in 1951, he realized that the "school belong[ed] to the goyim." There was a Jewish quota, and the few Jewish faculty lived as Christians. Nevertheless, he felt a greater sense of belonging than he had expected.[33] When Nuland decided to enter the surgery program, however, he realized he "faced discouraging odds against completing it." Only two of the thirteen interns would be chosen to be chief residents. Selection depended not just on ability but also on exhibiting the characteristics of a leader. And "there was another criterion as well, one openly discussed only among the few Jews who had made their way to the ascending levels of the pyramid. It was necessary to be a goy, and preferably Protestant. The last and only Jewish chief resident at Yale had been appointed in 1939, and it was no secret that he had abandoned his religion and was raising his children as Christians." But Nuland felt "a glimmer of hope." "One of the two chiefs taking over as I started my training was a very obviously Jewish-looking veteran of World War II named Ira Goldenberg."[34] I can only speculate about the extent to which Goldenberg felt like an outsider in 1969 and to what extent his "anomalous presence," in Nuland's words, contributed to his willingness to take positions at variance with those of many of his colleagues.

Klaus had studied nursing at the Hartford Hospital School of Nursing and Southern Connecticut State College. She was working as a private-duty nurse for one of the patients in the study and was eager for a new challenge when Wald invited her to join the research team. When she agreed, Wald expressed relief at being able share the burden of direct patient care.[35]

Although not officially a member of the research team, Donna Diers served as a consultant. After receiving an MS in nursing from Yale in 1964, she began teaching classes in research methods at the school. Later she earned a PhD from the University of Technology, Sydney, Australia. Although a pioneer in the use of large data sets in nursing research, she valued qualitative as well as quantitative methods. As a result, she was able to provide extensive help when Wald began to analyze the study findings.[36]

Wald credited the protest movements of the 1960s as well as Saunders with inspiring her to establish a new health care facility. As she commented to an interviewer, "It was the same month, almost to the day, when I heard Cicely Saunders, that Martin Luther King had the first march in Selma, Alabama."[37] By 1969 the antiwar, welfare rights, and women's movements had joined the civil rights movement. Wald noted that protest also reached medicine. Despite the passage of Medicare and Medicaid in 1965, health care activists continued to demand greater access. Some established neighborhood health centers (later community health centers) to provide primary health care to underserved areas. Funded by the federal government, the centers sought to promote broad social transformation and to empower patients to participate in their own medical care.[38] The holistic health movement insisted that patients be viewed as whole human beings, not simply the sum of their symptoms. The women's health movement criticized the technological focus of modern medicine and the enormous power physicians wielded over patients. Wald pointed to the resemblance between the natural childbirth and hospice movements, both of which criticized the medicalization of pivotal life events.[39] And many activists organized counter institutions to provide alternatives to established ones. Wald could look to food cooperatives, alternative newspapers, and free schools as models for the hospice she planned.[40]

Wald later stated that she had returned from her sabbatical at St. Christopher's Hospice in London "absolutely burning" to do something but feeling she "had come to the wrong city."[41] Even if she could not immediately find people interested in the hospice cause, however, New Haven in the late 1960s and early 1970s was a good place for a social activist. In 1967, a five-day insurrection in the Hill, an African American neighborhood, marked the beginning of widespread protest against the urban renewal projects that had destroyed many low-income and minority areas of the city.[42] The following year saw the establishment of the Hill Health

Center (now the Cornell Scott-Hill Health Center), the first federally funded neighborhood health center in Connecticut.[43] On May Day (May 1), 1970, thousands of people from all parts of the country gathered on the green to protest government attacks on the Black Panther Party.

Some social reform activity originated at Yale. Its chaplain was the famous civil rights and antiwar leader William Sloane Coffin, whom Wald called "the conscience of Yale."[44] He organized busloads to participate in the Mississippi Freedom Rides and later counseled Yale students on resisting the draft during the Vietnam War. As his biographer wrote, his arrest with Benjamin Spock and three others for protesting the Vietnam War in Washington, DC, in 1969 resulted in "one of the most celebrated trials of the decade."[45] Yale students played leadership roles in the American Independent Movement, a local organization that engaged in both antiwar and antiredevelopment causes, and founded several alternative institutions, including a school, a coffeehouse, and a printing press.[46]

Wald's study of dying people and their families took place against the background of those social change movements. "During the course of our original research," she later stated, "we were as apt to meet at vigils for peace, meetings in the black ghettoes of New Haven on behalf of their civil rights as we were in corridors, clinics, and meetings of the medical center."[47] She and Dobihal were especially active. Dobihal was arrested for antiwar protests with Coffin and Spock.[48] Diers recalled an early faculty meeting chaired by Wald that included a presentation on the Freedom Rides "with an appeal for us to join."[49] Diers also noted that Wald provided medical care during the May Day Panther rally and that she and Henry "joined anti-war marches whenever they could."[50]

Critiquing the American Way of Dying

The roots of the U.S. hospice movement can be found not only in Saunders's 1963 tour of the United States and the social ferment of the 1960s and 1970s but also in a long line of critics of the treatment of people at the end of life. A common assumption is that Kübler-Ross was the first to stress the importance of facing death openly and honestly and improving the quality of care of dying patients. Her 1969 book *On Death and Dying* argued that death had become a great taboo in our society, in part because the dying process was lonelier, more impersonal, and more dehumanized than ever before. Where once families gathered around the deathbed, dying patients now found themselves alone in ICUs, tethered to machines. The denial of mortality also reinforced the most "gruesome" features of death and dying. Unable to face their own anxieties, doctors prolonged life long after the hope of recovery had ended and failed to communicate honestly with the dying. Families hid behind falsely cheerful demeanors or withdrew entirely, thus heightening patients' sense of isolation. In addition, ICUs' regulations severely restricted the presence of relatives who wished to keep deathbed vigils. The remainder of the book, based on interviews with five hundred terminally ill hospital patients, presented Kübler-Ross's theory about the five emotional stages dying patients underwent (denial, anger, bargaining, depression, and acceptance).[51]

A past president of the American Medical Association declared Kübler-Ross "was a true pioneer in raising the awareness among the physician community and the general public about the important issues surrounding death [and] dying."[52] Other observers point to Kübler-Ross's originality by noting that *On Death and Dying* quickly became an international best seller, with more than a million copies purchased by 1976, and it has never been out of print.[53] But one historian reminds us that "books don't become best sellers because they are ahead of their time. They become best sellers when they tap into concerns that people are already mulling over, pull together ideas and data that have not yet spread beyond specialists and experts, and bring these all together in a way that is easy to understand and explain to others."[54] Writing in an unusually engaging and forceful style, Kübler-Ross popularized ideas that had circulated for at least a decade.

One of the first major U.S. books was Henry Feifel's 1959 *The Meaning of Death*, based on a symposium he organized at the American Psychological Association convention three years earlier.[55] "In the presence of death," Feifel wrote in his introduction, "Western culture, by and large, has tended to run, hide, and seek refuge in group norms and actuarial statistics. . . . Concern about death has been relegated to the tabooed territory heretofore occupied by diseases like tuberculosis and cancer and the topic of sex."[56] Essays by various psychologists, chaplains, and humanities scholars attempted to counter that taboo. Four years later, Jessica Mitford's *The American Way of Death* exposed the ways the funeral industry helped to convert mortality into a shameful secret.[57] The same year, Robert Fulton established the first seminar on death and dying at a major university.[58] In his edited volume *Death and Identity*, published in 1965, Fulton remarked that "research into grief and bereavement, studies of attitudes toward death, and recorded responses to death and dying have begun to appear in increasing plenitude in the social and medical science literature."[59]

Major sociological studies focused on the changes that had occurred in the care of dying patients since the end of World War II. Three books—Barney G. Glaser and Anselm L. Strauss's *Awareness of Dying* (1965) and *Time for Dying* (1968) and Jeanne C. Quint's *The Nurse and the Dying Patient* (1967)—were based on fieldwork collected at San Francisco Bay Area hospitals between 1961 and 1964. A fourth, *Passing On*, by David Sudnow, relied on nine months of observation at a county hospital and five months at a private facility between 1963 and 1965. Together, these texts described medical professionals who knew little about the emotional, social, and spiritual needs of the dying, felt extremely uncomfortable caring for that population, and tried to concentrate on patients most likely to recover.[60]

Bereaved family members were often far more caustic. A widow wrote in the January 1957 issue of the *Atlantic Monthly*, "There is a new way of dying today. It is the slow passage via modern medicine. If you are going to die it can prevent you from doing so for a very long time. To those who stand and watch, this seems like a ghastly imposition against God's will."[61] The author described her husband's harrowing hospital ordeal in lavish detail. A condensed version of the article appeared in *Reader's Digest* the following March, reaching a much larger audience.[62]

Theologians frequently protested against the terminal care that hospitals provided. In a prominent 1960 article in *Harper's*, for example, Joseph Fletcher, a professor at the Episcopal Theological School in Cambridge, Massachusetts, wrote that "medicine has a duty to relieve suffering equal to preserving life. Furthermore, it needs to re-examine its understanding of 'life' as a moral and spiritual good—not merely physical."[63] It is likely that Paul Ramsey had an especially important impact on Wald and the other researchers. In the 1968–69 academic year, he gave a series of distinguished lectures at the Yale Divinity School that were later published as a book titled *The Patient as Person: Explorations in Medical Ethics*. One chapter explored in depth the morality of giving both ordinary and extraordinary life-sustaining treatment to terminally ill patients.[64]

Many health professionals were acutely aware of the problems that sociologists, family members, and theologians exposed. By the late 1950s, articles in both national and state medical journals began to urge physicians to restore "dignity" to the dying. A major way was to focus less on prolonging life and more on improving its quality. A *New England Journal of Medicine* editorial quoted from the 1957 *Atlantic Monthly* essay by the widow condemning the "ghastly" new way of dying. The editors commented that the essay "should be required reading for physicians."[65] Writing in the *Journal of the American Medical Association*, Dr. Frank J. Ayd used nearly identical words when recommending the article to his colleagues.[66]

Many other doctors reiterated the essay's central argument. Edward H. Rynearson complained about the many cases of dying patients with intractable pain who were "kept alive indefinitely by means of tubes inserted into their stomachs, or into their veins, or into their bladders, or into their rectums."[67] A 1963 editorial in *Minnesota Medicine* declared, "We are now repeatedly faced with the question: how long and how heroically are we to attempt to defer death when there is no reasonable hope for recovery. . . .

Watching a *loved one* continue to suffer when repeated supportive or even drastic measures are required to keep him alive can be a heartbreaking ordeal."[68]

Physicians also encouraged their colleagues to interrogate their own attitudes toward mortality. "What would be the effect on medical education and the practice of medicine if significant numbers of physicians squarely faced their own deaths and accepted them?" John B. Graham asked rhetorically.[69] James A. Knight asserted, "A number of medical students and physicians have not worked through their own feelings about death and the finiteness of their own lives. Thus they cannot be comfortable with a patient as he approaches death."[70] And some doctors began to question practices of concealment. While many continued to argue that dying people could not bear to contemplate their mortality, a growing number contended that evasiveness served the needs of doctors more than those of patients.[71] According to Louis Lasagna, a professor of medicine and pharmacology at Johns Hopkins, the physician "often avoid[s] telling patients or relatives about imminent death" because his "ego and peace of soul are apt to be assaulted by the knowledge that he is unable to alter the downhill course. He may feel uncomfortable and ill at ease; he may also be so busy that he is reluctant to take the time required to get to know the patient and the family well enough to do the job properly."[72] Others noted that patients often intuited the seriousness of their conditions and that secrecy exacerbated their sense of loneliness and isolation.[73]

The concerns physicians raised had enormous relevance for nurses. Because they had the most sustained contact with dying patients, they often witnessed the suffering the new technologies inflicted.[74] Especially when they were convinced that doctors had kept patients alive primarily for research purposes, nurses often protested that death should have come sooner.[75] The onus of secrecy also fell on nurses. Patients often asked nurses to reveal the information their physicians had withheld.[76] Nevertheless, because doctors made the decisions about the withdrawal of treatment and the extent of disclosure, the writings by nurses focused on the care they themselves delivered.

Surveying the "Cumulative Indexes" of the *American Journal of Nursing* between 1900 and 1960, Jeanne C. Quint (later Benoliol) found "little evidence that care of the dying was ever a major concern of nurses in this country." The few articles listed focused overwhelmingly on technical issues, ignoring "the psychological aspects of care."[77] By the late 1950s, however, a growing number of essays in major nursing journals addressed that theme. Their dominant message differed dramatically from the one early twentieth-century nursing leaders delivered. Historian Barbara Melosh notes that although the first supervisors of student nurses "tacitly acknowledged students' emotions in the face of death," they insisted on self-control.[78] But now nurses warned that "composure strategies" too often led to avoidance of patients as death approached.[79] Drawing on the writings of a New York psychiatrist, Wilma R. Lewis asserted that if the nurse "can conquer her inclination to withdraw into starchy, impersonal efficiency in the face of her own anxieties about death and meet the patient on a human level, she may render an immeasurable service."[80]

"The Student's Page" in the *American Journal of Nursing* was replete with descriptions of initial encounters with death. Most named the patients and tried to understand them as whole people, with distinct emotional needs and life issues. An article titled "The Death of a Young Man" opened this way: "Mike was a 17-year-old, apparently healthy, high school senior. He played baseball, enjoyed parties and dates, planned to attend college, and was considered a big tease by his many friends and family of six."[81] Dorothy Whitehouse's article began, "As I walked into the ward, I glanced at the identification card on the foot of the fourth bed. 'Johnny, age 22 months.' There was more on the card but I did not read it just then; I was more interested in the little boy. He sat in the middle of the bed, sad-faced, clutching a small, blue, woolly rabbit."[82] And rather than emphasizing their struggles for control, most students stressed the closeness they achieved and the empathy and compassion they had conveyed. Mary L. Knipe realized that Mrs. C "needed to have people around who were able to just be there, not necessarily to talk, but to make her feel that she was not alone in the lonely process of dying."[83] Three other students were glad that a fourteen-year-old boy "had been able to unburden his fears and complaints in spite of his tendency to be apologetic when complaining."[84]

In short, more than a decade before the appearance of Kübler-Ross's landmark book, a host of academics, health professionals, and popular writers had begun to criticize medicine's overriding emphasis on recovery and cure, the secrecy surrounding dire diagnoses and prognoses, and the lack of attention to the needs of patients approaching finality. Those complaints occasionally were translated into action. In January 1969, oncologist Melvin J. Krant described a program established the previous year at Boston's Lemuel Shattuck's Hospital involving social workers, psychiatrists, and nurses who worked "as a team of experts with the physicians investigating patient and family needs and developing services . . . to ease the ache of dying and to offer support for the family." Krant emphasized that physicians must regard chronic illness and death "as being natural and inevitable" and "not distort the role of medicine into a top-heavy 'curative' priority."[85]

When *On Death and Dying* appeared in 1969, Wald and her colleagues studied it closely and repeatedly debated its findings. Kübler-Ross's visit to Yale the following year, when she interviewed two patients in Wald's study, generated enormous excitement. But the researchers drew on many other sources as well. Wald's notes specifically mentioned the works by Glaser and Strauss, a consultation with Quint, and a visit to Krant's project. As Wald indicated when she stated that Saunders "opened the door" during her tour, in 1963, American health professionals already were struggling with the issues Saunders had raised. Wald expected her study to provide the information she needed to create a hospice to address them.

2

Doctor and Nurse

When Wald brought together professionals from different disciplines to conduct her study, she envisioned them working as a group of equals. She also expected teamwork to be a vital component of the facility she planned to establish. As she frequently noted, the staff operated as a team at St. Christopher's, the London hospice that was her model. Moreover, many of the contemporary political movements she supported sought to disrupt hierarchical social arrangements.

Wald was especially eager to alter the traditional relationships between doctors and nurses. By 1969, the balance of power between them had begun to shift. We saw in the last chapter how Wald's mentor Peplau had argued that nurses could claim unique expertise by focusing on their personal relationships with patients. The expansion of high-tech medicine enabled nurses to enhance their status in another way. During the 1960s, ICUs and coronary care units increasingly contained new technologies such as defibrillators, feeding tubes, and respirators. Especially during the many hours when medical staff was unavailable, nurses in those units assumed responsibilities doctors previously had considered part of their exclusive domain.[1] As Wald explained, "The hospital is larger and more complicated and filled with equipment that requires many staff members with special skills and particular interests who are involved in a single patient's care."[2] She thus hoped to be able to work closely with many doctors at Yale New Haven Hospital (YNHH).

She soon realized, however, that very few hospital physicians understood the goals of her research and the role she expected to play. As a result, she decided that rather than relying on the entire medical staff to refer patients to her, she would select participants only from the rosters of the two doctors on her team. Because Wessel was a pediatrician and had very few terminally ill patients in his practice, her decision meant that Goldenberg, a breast cancer oncologist and surgeon, became the primary doctor in the study. Approximately three hundred patients visited his breast cancer clinic each year.[3]

Wessel noted that Wald worked best with Goldenberg. Their common experiences of being Jews at Yale may have strengthened their relationship. I have noted that Sherwin Nuland was surprised to find that the chief resident of Yale's surgical program in the early 1950s was the "very obviously Jewish-looking" Goldenberg. Anti-Semitism at Yale had greatly diminished by 1969, when Wald and Goldenberg began to work together. But when Wald attended the Yale School of Nursing in the late 1930s and early 1940s and when she returned first as a professor and then as a dean in the 1950s, she too may have been considered an outsider on an overwhelmingly Christian campus.[4]

Wald also must have felt that she had made the right choice because Goldenberg's views about hospital care for dying people seemed closely aligned with her own. In December 1968, he lambasted house staff who acted "almost as if there's something evil about being sick" and seemed to consider it a waste of time to care for dying patients. "This upsets me a great deal," he remarked.[5] At a conference with hospital staff the following year, he explained that "aloneness" was often the most serious problem of people at the very end of life: "If there's someone there just to be able to say a word or two, then I think we have met one of the great needs." He acknowledged that doctors often had to make a "conscious effort to screw up this courage and go into the room and just sit there for five minutes and talk to the patient and answer whatever

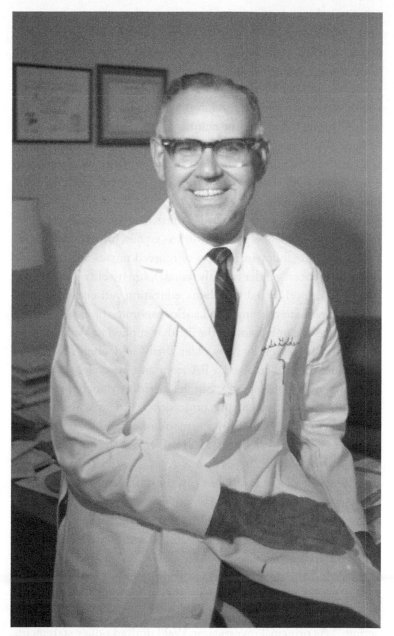

FIG. 2. Ira S. Goldenberg
(Credit: Yale University, Harvey Cushing/John Hay Whitney Medical Library)

questions the patient may have and give whatever support seems most appropriate." Nevertheless, he urged his colleagues not to avoid that task. He also demanded absolute honesty. "I have very, very strong feelings myself about lying to patients," he stated. "I think it is wrong." When patients ask if they are dying, physicians should answer truthfully, though they might want to add "indeed we're all going to die at some point, it's inevitable" and "we're going to keep you comfortable, we have medications available." Nurses who realized that patients had not been told what was happening must "button-hole the doctor involved, sit down and talk them him about the problem."[6]

Wald's personal characteristics must have bolstered her belief that she and Goldenberg could work as equals. One historian concluded that the following factors reinforced nurses' subordination in the late 1960s: "gender (mostly female), age (twenty-something), educational level (usually diploma education rather than college and postgraduate training), and socioeconomic status as nurses."[7] Gender was the only item on the list that applied to Wald. In 1969, she was fifty-two, eight years older than Goldenberg. Instead of a diploma, she had received a BA from an elite college and MAs from two major universities. She had held extremely prestigious positions within the nursing profession. And as a woman, she derived her status partly from the men in her family. Her husband was an engineer and architect. Her brother was the eminent Princeton historian Carl E. Schorske.

Moreover, Wald's leading role in the study demanded that she receive more respect and autonomy than doctors typically accorded members of her profession. "One characteristic essential to any researcher is independence in thought," she wrote in 1964, "yet traditionally the nurse's role has been passive rather than creative. It is usual that the doctor diagnoses and prescribes while the nurse carries out his orders. This pattern of relationship is antithetical to the nurse scientist who must observe for herself and devise ways of acting."[8] As principal investigator, Wald drafted policy statements, gained intimate knowledge of the study participants, ran the team's meetings, and analyzed the findings.

Interviewed in 2016 about her experience on the study, Klaus emphasized the novelty of attending meetings with physicians who treated her as a colleague rather than as an underling. She also recalled Wald and Goldenberg as two highly respected individuals who appreciated and listened to each other.[9] Nevertheless, they frequently clashed. Soon after Goldenberg assumed his more prominent position on the research team, Wald asked whether they should ever "deviate from the hierarchical system" or "toy around with consensus." He responded that a clear leadership structure was essential. Federal regulations mandated that neighborhood health centers make decisions collectively. Goldenberg pointed to the deleterious consequences at the recently opened Hill Health Center: "Every single decision is made, whether the john is going to be cleaned or to buy yellow soap or white soap is made by consensus. The center is in shambles right now because nobody recognizes that consensus does not work—you need to have somebody in charge." He also made it clear that he intended to be that person. Although Wald could work closely with him in caring for his patients, he was "unalterably opposed" to sharing authority with her. He acknowledged that she had overall responsibility for the research project and that he could only advise her in that domain. But he also insisted that whenever she rejected his advice, she had to tell him why.[10]

Goldenberg could make those demands not only because he was a physician but also because Wald regarded him as indispensable. She could think of no other YNHH doctor who shared so many of her views about terminal care. Moreover, the project was far more important to her than to him, and she worried constantly that he would lose interest. If he withdrew, the study would end. Her fears heightened when the research group began to discuss the development of the hospice. He initially expressed enormous enthusiasm about the project. When he began to waver, she realized how essential his support was. He was a "powerful person" with "connections all over." It was thus vital that the group had him "on board."[11]

Ironically, Goldenberg was able to use his close connection to patients, which Wald highly valued, to justify his requirements for participation in the study. If his views about terminal care diverged sharply from those of his colleagues, he resembled other doctors of his time in his paternalism. He argued that he knew what was best for his patients because he understood their personal lives, not only their diseases. According to notes of a meeting held soon after he assumed a more prominent role in the study, his major fear was that "Mrs. Wald may interject herself between him and his patients. As it is now, he is social worker, visiting nurse, bon vivant, and many other functions and they are all rooted in the patient-physician relationship. He does not want this destroyed." In response to a question from the dean of the school of nursing about whether women with breast cancer felt comfortable discussing sensitive issues with a man, he stated that patients did not hesitate to talk to him, even about "some of the most delicate subjects [that] revolve around sex." He also asserted that his close relationship to patients had therapeutic value. "I am firmly of the opinion that my medications do a certain amount of good," he remarked, "but the psychological support that the patient gets from her physician is as important, if not more important than any medicines that I give, and I am firmly convinced that a lot of these people live longer just because of the support they get and nothing more."[12] Many months later, when Wald recommended that a patient receive a tranquilizer before undergoing a difficult procedure, he responded that his "own soothing voice is enough."[13] Still later, when Goldenberg learned that a family had written to Wald, thanking her for the care she had provided a patient in her last weeks, he remarked that he usually was the recipient of such letters.

Wald's difficulties conferring with Goldenberg were emblematic of their relationship. Although they had agreed to meet regularly to discuss cases, he rarely made time to do so. When she told him after one of his clinics that she hoped they could sit down and talk, he said he had to leave immediately for another appointment. Wald then asked if she could walk with him but felt "a little bit angry that he couldn't even give me five minutes of his time." When he agreed, she dropped her belongings, knowing she would have to return for them, and "tagged along with this sense of irritation in me."[14] Wald described her experience preparing to attend the clinic on another occasion: "I began to feel that he was going to be critical about something, and I found myself cleaning my shoes and washing my dress again, and ironing it and concerned that my nurses' hat was unkempt. I thought to myself I should get a new hat and be neat and tidy and so forth." Her behavior seemed more appropriate for encountering "a nursing supervisor who was particularly strict about clothes" than for meeting a colleague.[15] She considered herself partly to blame. A few years earlier, she had quoted with approval a Columbia Teachers' College dissertation that concluded that "nurses in the hospital, both collectively and individually, reinforce and strengthen [traditional] stereotypes in their attitudes and behavior toward different categories of professional workers." Accepting their "minor role," nurses performed "rituals of obeisance" to staff they considered their superiors.[16] Wald thus berated herself for being "so uptight" before encountering Goldenberg.[17]

She appears to have been relieved to learn she was not alone in her feelings. The nurses in his clinic confided that they too were "very uptight," constantly trying to please Goldenberg and afraid of his criticism.[18] Additional feedback came from Maddy Gerrish, the social worker in a program for terminally ill cancer patients at Boston's Lemuel Shattuck Hospital, who visited Wald. At both a dinner party at Wald's house and a research meeting the following morning, Gerrish observed Goldenberg closely. Later she reported that she had seen him "intimidating and attacking" others. Wald also discussed Goldenberg frequently with Donna Diers. She too described Goldenberg as arrogant and abrasive. Both Gerrish and Diers added, however, that if Wald adopted a more confrontational stance, she might find that he was less powerful than she assumed.[19] As we will see, she eventually was able to influence Goldenberg's stance on one critical issue but was not on many others.

Although Wald never felt comfortable with Goldenberg, she began to focus less on her troubles with him and more on his relationships with patients. She later noted that when she had asked for recommendations of doctors who took a special interest in patients, Goldenberg's name repeatedly emerged.[20] His warm and close connection to his patients impressed her too, and she often recorded their effusive comments. "Oh, what a doctor!" one woman exclaimed. "I mean here's a doctor who's a human being, you don't see many of these. He has love, compassion, patience. He doesn't even like to have patients wait like other doctors. They don't care."[21] Klaus's observation of Goldenberg's conversation with one of his patients in a nursing home also must have impressed Wald. The woman was "miserable" and asked if she needed a private-duty nurse because she had received so little attention. "He pulled up a chair and had a leisurely visit with the patient. She obviously was distressed, and she had written down a list of complaints so she wouldn't forget anything. . . . He allowed her plenty of time to explain her problems and encouraged her to elaborate on them. He examined her physically and told her he would do something about each problem, and that he and I would discuss it. Her spirits seemed improved after the visit." Klaus added that "when we got to the nurses station, Dr. Goldenberg admitted he had a gut reaction to the patient. He said he didn't care for her whining personality which was nothing new. She had also been this way before she had gotten so sick. I must comment that he couldn't have been more considerate of her needs when he was in the room with the patient."[22]

But Wald did not approve of all aspects of Goldenberg's relationships. Despite his claim that he never abandoned patients close to death, he seemed to disappear when his patients were actively dying. Nurses who needed orders for oxygen and pain medication for patients in extremis were told he was unavailable. Wald was especially stunned when he failed to respond to requests for a woman to whom he had "a very close attachment." She had been his patient for many years, and in his office, he prominently displayed the large ceramic dog she had given him.[23] Nevertheless, he ignored the messages Wald and Klaus left with his administrative assistant throughout the day. One of the few times he attended a death was when the end came suddenly and he happened to be in the patient's room. Wald also accused him of favoring patients who were white, nonimmigrant, affluent, and college educated. Although he adamantly insisted that socioeconomic status never influenced the way he cared for his patients, she observed him selecting women with privileged backgrounds to participate in the study, recognizing their symptoms sooner than those of others, and spending more time with them.

Secrecy

Wald's most serious criticism was that Goldenberg hid bad news. Although he preached the importance of honesty, his practices often diverged sharply from his prescription. He disclosed cancer diagnoses but employed various strategies to conceal grim prognoses. Wald learned the hard way that Goldenberg ignored problems that indicated advanced disease that could not be fixed. During one clinic visit, she asked a woman if she wanted to repeat her question about her swollen arm, which had remained unanswered. After the appointment ended, "Dr. G. proceeded to say—'Never bring up in front of a patient a question like that. There is nothing that I can answer about the arm and all it does is to make her feel helpless and hopeless.' I explained to Dr. G. that what I had been trying to do was to help her ask any questions that she had already raised herself and that I wasn't putting new ideas into her head. He then reiterated, '*Never* do that again.'"[24] When Goldenberg answered questions about symptoms, he often minimized their significance. Thus he reassured one woman that her respiratory problems stemmed from a bad cold, although he believed the cause was liver metastasis. He knew a second woman's laryngitis meant she was "in real trouble" but "tried to play it down."[25] And he sought to persuade women who were close to death that recovery still was possible. After he told one woman she might go home in a few days, Wald left the room with him "and walking down the corridor, I asked if he really thought that she would go home, and he said no, he felt that she was slipping rather fast."[26]

In one case, Goldenberg repeatedly delayed diagnostic tests he believed would indicate disease progression. Born in 1912, Sofia Marsh had graduated from teacher training school in 1936. After caring for numerous family members—including her mother, her husband, her husband's mother, her father, and her sister—she was diagnosed with cancer. By the fall of 1970, the disease had spread to her bones, and she no longer could work. She lived with her daughter, a graduate student engaged to be married. Klaus, her primary nurse, phoned Goldenberg in December to inform him that Marsh had experienced a great deal of pain. He responded that she might need an X-ray to discover the cause but they should wait to see if the pain subsided. He later told Klaus that he believed the test would reveal that her condition had worsened. Shortly afterwards, Marsh left for California with a friend. After a bad fall there, she had an X-ray, which indicated she had a lesion on her skull. When Klaus conveyed that news to Goldenberg in January 1970, he told her that Marsh should not worry and he would see her the next week. It is not clear whether Marsh mentioned the suspicious X-ray on that visit, but Goldenberg told Klaus that he purposely avoided the test because if he found evidence of a new metastasis he would have to tell her about it, and he did not want to do that. At the end of the month, Marsh complained about a heavy hangover from medication, which Klaus was convinced indicated "cerebral involvement" but knew she should not mention. A few days later, Marsh asked Klaus why Goldenberg had not ordered the blood test that she usually had every six months and was now overdue. When Klaus transmitted the question to Goldenberg, he replied that he had purposely ignored the test because he believed it would show that Marsh's illness had advanced, and he did not want her to know. In the middle of February, Klaus reported that Marsh experienced substantial pain. Goldenberg again decided to do nothing, explaining that the patient usually phoned him directly when she was worried and he would wait for her call. If he pushed information on her, he would just make her more upset. By then, she had had a liver function test, which, he admitted to Klaus, revealed very serious involvement. "But don't dare tell her," he instructed.[27] On March 15, Marsh did have the X-rays she had requested four months earlier. As anticipated, they showed that the disease had spread, and she underwent radiation and surgery. Nevertheless, her health continued to deteriorate. Soon after moving to a nursing home in July, she finally learned the results of the liver test. She died the following month.

Treatment near the end of life sometimes represented another form of obfuscation. Wald recalled hearing Goldenberg recommend Geritol over the phone.[28] At the end of the call, he explained, "It gives her something to do." After prescribing an antibiotic to another woman, he again commented, "It gives her something to do," adding, "not that I think it's going to accomplish anything."[29] When the suggested therapy was radiation, as it often was, the consequences could be serious. To be sure, Goldenberg believed radiation sometimes had therapeutic benefits, even when patients were extremely ill. "There can be little doubt," he wrote in 1966, "that assiduous [radiation] treatment of women with advanced breast cancer pays dividends in comfort as well as increased longevity for the afflicted patient."[30] Nevertheless, evidence indicates that he urged some women with late-stage disease to undergo radiation even when he had little faith it would help. A forty-six-year-old clerical worker married to a factory foreman, Janet Fischer earned the affection of the entire nursing staff during her many admissions to YNHH. When she returned at the end of July 1969, Goldenberg suggested her husband begin to prepare the children for the inevitable. At the same time, Goldenberg stated that he wanted her to have a month of brain radiation. A handwritten note Wald attached to the typed report read, "Dr. informs me doubts intervention."[31] It is unclear why Fischer consented. Her husband remarked that when she learned she needed radiation, "she just groaned and dreaded it." On her last admission, she had been treated "like a hide of beef." The staff had treated her roughly and hurt her terribly.[32] Since then the disease had spread to her hips, which made any movement even more painful. But Goldenberg could be very persuasive. Another patient noted that she had decided to have no more treatments, especially not brain radiation, until Dr. Goldenberg talked her into it.[33] Fischer was relieved to find that this time the staff treated her with greater sensitivity than they had on previous occasions. She also liked the radiologist, although he warned her that the type of radiation could cause brain damage. Goldenberg too worried about side effects. When Fischer suddenly became unresponsive a few days after treatment began, he feared it might have caused a cerebral hemorrhage. When she regained consciousness, radiation resumed, although she complained it made her feel "crazy."[34] She died on August 20, three weeks after her first radiation session.

We can understand Goldenberg's evasions and deceptions in various ways. Several commentators argue that doctors tend to experience a sense of personal failure when patients die.[35] Goldenberg explained why that feeling was especially intense among surgeons: "A patient's death is a defeat of something that we've done with our hands. Quite different from internists who talk about medication and can sort of sit with their arms akimbo. But we surgeons are there, we're dropping a scalpel, we're maneuvering, and it's quite an admission of defeat for our own handiwork."[36] Moreover, because he was an oncologist as well as a surgeon, he remained involved with patients after he operated, often trying one remedy after another before admitting defeat. Concealing information may have helped him gain at least the illusion of mastery over a situation he could not control. Day after day, he struggled with a disease that was depicted as a group of cells multiplying relentlessly and that was often fatal regardless of his best efforts. Historian and physician Barron H. Lerner recalled that when his doctor father feared that his wife's breast cancer had returned, he kept his anxiety to himself. "Although he had done what he could to ensure that my mother would receive excellent care," Lerner wrote, "beyond that, the situation was out of his control. . . . Yet staying in control—or appearing to—was what my father believed he needed to do, for his own sake and for others'. So he controlled what he could: information."[37]

Goldenberg may have had a similar motivation. If he could not stop the irresistible march of death, he could at least try to exert control by withholding grim news from patients. Some kinds of concealment enabled him to avoid confronting their most powerful and unruly emotions. He explained to Wald why he often became irritated when patients cried: "It depends on what they're crying about. If they're crying about something that we can take action on—either to give them medication or radiation or to do something about, then I think we're in great shape." But when they cried "out of desperation," he felt overwhelmed and had no idea how to respond.[38] On the few occasions when he felt he had to break bad news, he indicated that he approached the task with dread; it would "take guts," he said, to tell a woman with young children that death was near. Before he informed an elderly woman she was dying, he asked Wald to be present to help handle the outpouring of emotion he anticipated. Because he had "tried to hold off on letting her know exactly what is going on," the truth was "going to hit her like a boom."[39]

If Goldenberg sought to shield himself from the most intense pain and anguish his patients expressed, he did not try to distance himself entirely. Sociologist Larry Hirschhorn argued that professions "provide their members with professional 'armor,' with techniques and rules of action that allow them to minimize their emotional and psychological involvement with their clients. . . . Professional codes sanction such distance on the grounds that excessive identification can limit the professional's capacity to give help."[40] But Goldenberg prided himself on his close bonds with patients and his empathy for their suffering. It is possible that he occasionally lied to himself as well as others to keep his sorrow at bay. Goldenberg's administrative assistant explained why his reports in patients' charts were often more favorable than their conditions warranted. "Because he got so upset when his patients became sick," she had encouraged him "to look on the bright side of things."[41] Optimism also helped to sustain his relationships with patients. As sociologist Nicholas A. Christakis wrote, good news was "pleasant to deliver" and "generally unthreatening to the physician-patient relationship."[42] "Isn't he a wonderful doctor?" Fischer remarked after Goldenberg promised radiation would prove beneficial. "He works so hard and has such confidence."[43] When asked why he assured a woman close to death that she soon would be on her feet, he responded that he told her what she wanted to hear. Finally, it is important to note that Goldenberg was following customary practices. In their classic study of YNHH in 1968, Raymond S. Duff and August B. Hollingshead wrote that "information regarding the probable prognosis of a severe disease . . . was guarded even more carefully by the professionals than was the diagnosis."[44] Barney G. Glaser and Anselm L. Strauss found a similar reluctance to reveal the approach of death among the doctors at Oakland and San Francisco hospitals in the early 1960s. Like Goldenberg, many doctors emphasized the importance of trying to "do something" and "*act[ed]* as though they were still trying to save the patient's life."[45] Even today studies consistently find that although doctors are far more willing than their predecessors to disclose disturbing diagnoses, the great majority continue to hide grave prognoses.[46]

Patients varied in their responses to Goldenberg's practices of concealment. Some accepted his reassurance. Wald often observed women leave his office relieved and happy after he had given them what she knew to be misleading information. Others, however, were more skeptical. Wald described Ellen Black as a "very neatly dressed, attractive white-haired woman." She had worked as an office administrator for many years until illness forced her to quit. Now she "staggered" and "trembled" when she walked.[47] Klaus was with her when Goldenberg promised she could return to work in a few months. She responded, "Oh, you must be out of your mind."[48] A few days later, Klaus wrote that Black "asked Dr. Goldenberg very directly, 'what do you think we can expect in the way of improvement?' Dr. Goldenberg said laughingly, 'Oh, you should be up walking around like a young chick real soon again.' I think she took this with a grain of salt. She didn't smile as he said it, but really studied his face for the truth."[49] Klaus commented that Black's bones were so poor it was unlikely she ever would walk again. When Black realized she was dying, two months before the date Goldenberg had set for her return to the office, she angrily told a nurse to inform him "his schedules were a little bit off."[50]

Some patients reacted differently at different times. Annie Durand had received a radical mastectomy in 1961. When the disease returned in 1966, she had undergone hormonal treatment and chemotherapy. Despite those treatments, she was extremely ill by the fall of 1970. Her husband had taken over the housework. The son living at home had reduced his hours at work to be able to provide more nursing care. And the entire family anxiously awaited the return of the other son, who had been given a special leave by the Army to see his mother before she died. After visiting the home in early November, Klaus wrote that the patient "seemed a bit skeptical of her future course and didn't accept Dr. Goldenberg's encouragement with much faith."[51] At the beginning of December, however, she was "very relieved with Dr. Goldenberg's encouragement."[52] Later that month, Durand seemed very short of breath when she walked into the clinic, and she complained about double vision. Although Goldenberg did not respond to her question about that new symptom, "she seemed quite encouraged on leaving the clinic, having received good support from Dr. Goldenberg."[53] But when her condition sharply deteriorated, she again became more distrustful. Visiting the home in January 1971, Klaus observed that even with her husband's help the patient had to "struggle" to get to the bathroom. Now Klaus tried to offer reassurance, telling Durand that Goldenberg "has many more treatments or tricks in the bag to help her with." She "appreciated the encouragement" but took it "with a grain of salt."[54] She also refused to believe Goldenberg when he informed her that the results of her recent cardiogram were "'ginger peachy, A-OK,' and not to worry."[55] The following day, she consulted an intern, who admitted they had found an abnormality. "So there was something," Durand remarked. "I guess Dr. Goldenberg didn't want to worry me."[56] She died a month later.

Goldenberg's attempts to camouflage critical information were a frequent topic of conversation among Wald, Klaus, and Diers. They too had various reactions. All three had read the growing literature about the harmful effects of medical concealment and expressed a commitment to honesty. But Diers and Klaus were far more likely than Wald to justify Goldenberg's actions. Diers, for example, argued that his decision to tell Black she soon would be able to work "may be in a way an awfully good technique of his, even though we find it quite offensive. Because it does give the patient time to adjust to the fact that she may not be able to go back to teaching as she becomes aware of the fact that her body is going to deteriorate."[57] Perhaps because the task of concealing grim information frequently fell to Klaus, she had the most complicated response. She had felt extremely uncomfortable misleading Marsh and Durand and had done so only because she had been trained to follow doctors' instructions. She also argued that had Marsh learned the results of her X-ray earlier, she might have begun treatment when it still was likely to have some benefit. But Klaus also gave Goldenberg the benefit of the doubt, pointing out that he knew Marsh better than they did. And there was at least some indication that he made the correct call in that case. Marsh had admitted that she "didn't like to pin Dr. Goldenberg too precisely" and refrained from asking about the possibility of liver involvement until a month before she died. Even then, according to Klaus, she "stated that she doesn't want to know every detail at this stage and purposely doesn't ask Dr. Goldenberg everything."[58] Whenever she began to ask if she was near the end, she "rattled on about something else." She "really didn't want to know," Klaus concluded.[59]

Klaus also had come to believe Goldenberg might have treated Fischer appropriately. One morning Fischer had been extremely depressed, saying she never would go home again and was a burden on everyone. Klaus had had no encouragement to offer, "and things looked really poor at that time." But "Dr. Goldenberg came in full of energy and confidence and said, 'well, we're going to start radiation for about four weeks and maybe in two weeks you'll be strong enough to go home.' When he walked out, I was kind of thinking, 'hmmm, what did he say that for?' But she was so happy at this little speck of hope, so I felt as if I was handling it wrong."[60]

Wald's allegiance to honesty never wavered. Although she occasionally found herself violating her principles, she never condoned her lapses. Thus she chastised herself when she realized she had used euphemisms, telling a woman on the verge of death that she was "convalescing" or omitting the words "cancer" and "dying" when explaining the purpose of her study. She frequently noted that people needed the truth to be able to grow emotionally and make practical arrangements. Marsh, for example, might have advanced the date of her daughter's wedding had she understood how close she was to death. Although Wald agreed everyone needed hope, she argued that hope should be realistic. A woman who had hoped to travel to Europe might find herself looking forward to a special restaurant meal with her husband instead. Wald also acknowledged that she was not qualified to assess many of Goldenberg's medical decisions. Nevertheless, she was especially censorious when he urged patients with late stages of disease to undergo radiation. Radiation not only fostered false hopes but also consumed time people could better spend getting ready for death. It also precipitated new problems. Wald pointed specifically to brain radiation, citing Fischer, who had not wanted that treatment but was told it might benefit her.

Research

The sharpest conflicts occurred when Wald believed Goldenberg recommended intensive treatments to serve the interests of medical researchers more than of patients. Goldenberg was actively involved in the research enterprise at Yale Medical School. His 1968 curriculum vitae listed seventy-nine articles in medical journals.[61] One unusually well-documented case demonstrates Wald's response to his attempts to negotiate between his concerns as an investigator and as a physician. Ruth Cohen was in her early forties when she joined Wald's study. The wife of a lawyer, Cohen had undergone a mastectomy seven years earlier; when the cancer metastasized, her local oncologist had administered further treatments. By November 1969, however, he had nothing more to offer and thus sent her to Goldenberg. She quickly became one of his favorite patients. He described her as a "charming, intelligent woman, with extremely fine insight into her problem and all that is going on."[62] She also impressed Wald. Soon the two women discovered that they had many friends and acquaintances in common. It also is possible that both Wald and Goldenberg felt a special sense of kinship with Cohen because all three were Jewish. Wald noted that Cohen received "quite a bit of attention" from the entire clinic staff. Nurses as well as doctors hovered around her.[63]

Cohen's special status in the clinic could not compensate for the hopelessness of her situation. She told Goldenberg's assistant that for the first time she felt "the buggers are going to get me instead of me getting the buggers" and complained to Goldenberg that "the rat poison now didn't seem to be doing any good."[64] Goldenberg seemed equally disheartened. At the end of his long clinic day, he commented that his medications offered little help to many patients; a case in point was Ruth Cohen, who was rapidly approaching death.[65]

But there was one more option. At the end of December, Goldenberg announced that Cohen would undergo a hypophysectomy, the surgical removal of the pituitary gland. Although rarely performed today, the operation often was used in the past for temporary control of advanced breast cancer.[66] Rachel Carson, for example, had suffered from the disease for several years by 1963, when her doctor, George Crile Jr., recommended she receive the surgery. Although a cardiologist warned that Carson's serious heart condition would make the procedure especially dangerous, she had exhausted all other remedies and finally consented, flying from her home in Washington, DC, to the Cleveland Clinic where Crile could supervise her care. The operation took place on March 18. Such a desperate measure might seem totally out of character for Carson as well as her doctor. She had repeatedly expressed her wish for a peaceful end. Crile had often railed against the use of aggressive actions for gravely ill patients. And both had preached the need to accept the inevitable. In the event, however, neither could refuse one final attempt to avert death. Carson survived the operation, but she remained critically ill, experiencing heart irregularities as well as jaundice from liver metastases. She flew home on April 6 and died eight days later.[67]

In Cohen's case as well, a hypophysectomy represented a last ditch effort. The doctor who performed her procedure was William F. Collins Jr., professor and chief of neurosurgery at Yale University School of Medicine and neurosurgeon in chief at YNHH. Because numerous patients had received the surgery, it could not be considered experimental. But Collins had studied various techniques for performing the operation since 1955, and it is thus likely that he viewed Cohen as a research subject as well as a patient.[68] According to Wald's account, "Dr. Goldenberg explained that the lesion on Cohen's breast and extending across her chest wall is coming out of control to such a degree that he feels he has nothing else he can offer her so last Wednesday when Mrs. Cohen came into the clinic, he, Dr. Collins, Mr. and Mrs. Cohen decided on this procedure."[69] We have no way of knowing what kind of information the Cohens received and to what extent they participated in the decision. Largely in response to reports of the abuse of human subjects, the federal government soon would begin to require investigators to obtain informed consent from patients.[70] At the end of 1969, however, both the government and universities still deferred to investigators' judgment about what constituted ethical practice. Dr. Collins may have been especially persuasive. In an article published six months earlier, he and his colleague wrote that only two of the hundred patients they had studied had refused the surgery.[71]

Goldenberg had warned in 1964 that a hypophysectomy was "not something for the occasional surgeon to perform and even in the most skilled hands morbidity and mortality may be considerable."[72] Now, however, he told Wald that although he "was not certain whether or not the procedure will discourage the growth of the lesions . . . it can do no harm."[73] When talking to Cohen, he downplayed any pain and suffering the procedure might involve, assuring her that she would not need a private-duty nurse. Was he persuaded by a recent article in which Collins and his colleagues claimed that a new technique meant the "discomfort and risk" of the operation were "small"?[74] Or was Goldenberg, like Crile, willing to try almost anything that possibly could help a desperately ill (and especially favored) patient?

Visiting Cohen the day before the surgery, Wald learned that Collins planned to insert a tiny instrument through Cohen's nasal passage. Because the chance of damage to the optic nerve was high, Collins would take frequent X-rays. In addition, Cohen would have to be awake enough to report whether she had any double vision. Finding that Cohen had a "tremendous amount of anxiety," Wald offered to accompany her throughout the procedure and act as her nurse.[75] As a result, Wald was able not only to perform an invaluable personal service but also to describe the operation in considerable detail.

The surgery was scheduled for eight thirty, but Wald and Cohen were not admitted into the operating room until noon. In the interim, they waited in a "very, very tiny space," observing "much coming and going back and forth [with] people very tense and involved." In addition to Collins, the staff included another doctor, an electronic engineer, and two nurses. A sociable woman, Cohen "kept trying to keep them at ease" by raising various subjects that might interest them, but they remained focused on "all the instruments." The procedure began by putting "a circle around the head and inject[ing] screws above each eyebrow and to the back of the head." The patient then had to "lay absolutely still on a bare table" while the doctors inserted larger and larger tubes into her nostrils. "The grinding and the noise . . . went on for three hours and then huge machines were brought in to freeze the pineal body, so that the room became so encumbered with machines that it was . . . very macabre and then every 5 to 10 minutes we all would have to leave the room and leave her alone while x-rays were being taken." Although Wald was allowed to administer more sedation,

Cohen "became so white that at times I almost thought she was about to expire and at one point, I didn't even feel I could hold her hand anymore, because I was afraid that she would realize how upset I was." Soon Cohen began to retch. When Dr. Collins finally released the screws on her head, "blood was dripping down either side of her temple." After most people had left the room, a nurse shrieked. The patient "was lying with blood spewing from her mouth and from the two spots down her temple, her face was white." Wald suddenly saw that she "had had a crown of thorns. This had been her Christmas Eve halo."[76]

If Wald sometimes hesitated to confront Goldenberg, she had no trouble doing so here. Meeting Wald and Cohen as soon as they left the operating room, he asserted that the surgery had been very successful, by which he meant there had been no complications. Wald commented, "You sure ought to get a fur coat for this procedure."[77] Since the 1950s, critics had charged that doctors prescribed unnecessary surgery for financial gain; the purchase of a fur coat was understood to refer to that accusation. Wald thus suggested that Goldenberg had allowed mercenary motives to influence his consent to Cohen's operation.[78]

Cohen burst into tears when she returned to her room and saw her husband. She then slept until the following morning. Wald arrived home "extremely upset."[79] For a brief time, Goldenberg continued to minimize Cohen's experience, claiming that she had been laughing rather than crying when she returned to her hospital room.[80] But he soon admitted that "it is a very traumatic experience and it takes a very stoic individual who has got a lot of sedation, and no matter how much is given, it is not enough."[81] Despite his earlier assertion that Cohen would not need a special nurse, he said he was glad Wald had acted in that role and did not believe any patient could have endured such a "catastrophic procedure" without "somebody to hang on to."[82] He also acknowledged his colleagues had not viewed Mrs. Cohen "as a functioning, reacting human being."[83] Especially when procedures were performed under local anesthesia, "there has to be some warmth."[84] And he expressed relief when she was moved to a general medicine floor, where the staff were less "gung-ho" and much more sensitive than the neurosurgeons he knew.[85]

Although Wald had initially shared Goldenberg's admiration for Cohen, familiarity gradually bred contempt. Early in 1970, Wald decided Cohen had a "life of superficiality." She "seemed to have everything in the world," but it was all "tinsel."[86] No longer a sign of her good taste, Cohen's exquisite outfits increasingly were viewed as a symbol of her vanity and shallowness: "Every time she has had problems that she has had to deal with, she has taken them to Elizabeth Arden or [bought] beautiful clothes."[87] As a result, Wald concluded, Cohen lacked the capacity to deal with her looming death.

But Wald also grieved when Cohen no longer was able to keep up appearances. After seeing her at Goldenberg's clinic on February 4, 1970, five weeks after the operation, Wald wrote that the decline was "very painful" to see. The woman who had "been immaculately dressed, beautifully, always socially poised" was now "almost on her knees." Her body "looked limp and bedraggled."[88] Wald was thus appalled when she learned that Cohen soon would enter Hunter 5, the ward for patients in research studies, where Collins would study the aftereffects of the hypophysectomy. That was standard procedure. Collins wrote that he admitted most hypophysectomy patients to the hospital at two and six month intervals after surgery.[89]

Wald erupted in fury when she learned about the plan, stating that she "hate[d] Dr. Collins" and that Cohen would be subjected to procedures that had no therapeutic potential. Although Goldenberg insisted that the interests of patient and researcher coincided, she remained unconvinced. Wald also noted that she previously had tried to work with the Hunter 5 staff and found them adamantly opposed to her philosophy of palliative care. With Cohen's time running out, Wald insisted her comfort must be the only concern.[90]

Cohen, however, had high hopes when she entered Hunter 5. Although she might have been inclined not to trust Goldenberg's assurances, he was able to convince her that the ward was "a very nice place." Despite her prior experience with Collins, she expected he "will help her so that she'll be able to go dancing on her own."[91] Various recent studies provide evidence of the "therapeutic misconception," the widespread belief of research subjects that treatment decisions are made solely on the basis of their individual health needs.[92] Before the implementation of informed consent, patients must have been especially prone to that misunderstanding. Cohen later would remark that patients should be told what to expect before all hospital procedures.[93]

Cohen's optimism quickly faded. Three days after arriving, she called Wald at home, complaining that the doctors and nurses had treated her solely as a "statistic." Although she had not slept for two nights, they had refused sedation for the following night on the grounds that the medication would interfere with scheduled tests. Wald readily agreed that the doctors had little interest in patient needs. After visiting Cohen later that day, Wald wrote, "They had really not given her an accurate description of what was going to happen to her. They said, oh, there would be just a few tests. In actuality the day before she'd had nothing by mouth." When the doctor arrived, he "said, 'OK, I'm ready to do the blood work now' and wheeled in a great big cart filled with test tubes and a large bottle and other equipment and arranged her to start drawing the blood giving no explanation to her or to [her nurse] as to what was going to happen and then he went out of the room and left her for 40 minutes while she stared at this rack of test tubes." When they tried to take blood, they had difficulty because one arm was swollen and her veins were fragile. The doctor spoke to her "very perfunctorily, said there's nothing to this test, and anger began to well up inside of her." Cohen confided that "she didn't really see what good this was doing her and she was beginning to feel it was all for posterity and she wasn't interested in posterity." She could not take it anymore and demanded to leave.[94]

Klaus cared for Cohen during her week on Hunter 5, and she made a similar report: Cohen "was told the tests would be done a certain day, and the time schedules were off. Like, 'You will have the test done at 9 o'clock, and we will be through at 10:00, and at 10:00 you will eat breakfast,' and they didn't show up until 10:30, and she was starving, and she was weak and undergoing rigorous tests until about 12:30 or 1:00 o'clock on several days, and she was getting increasingly irritated, and these tests were exhausting."[95]

Cohen also had a lengthy visit from Bruce Fabric, a medical student briefly associated with Wald's project. According to his account, Cohen complained that although Collins was in charge of her care, he had visited her only once. The rest of the time, she saw only his laboratory assistants, one of whom had dirt on his fingernails that she assumed was blood from the test he administered to her or from his work in the lab. Either way it was a "gruesome image." Fabric could not imagine trying to fall asleep in that "chamber of horrors."[96]

Goldenberg initially downplayed Cohen's complaints, arguing that her lack of sleep was not a problem, she exaggerated her difficulties, and it was not urgent to move her to another ward or send her home. He also criticized her as childish for removing from her door a sign requesting nothing by mouth, an action Wald had applauded.[97] But once again, he gradually accepted Wald's version of events. At a meeting of Wald's research team, he asserted that he thought "clinical research can be done if the individual doing it recognizes that the person is indeed a person, and is not a laboratory animal." Cohen's management "was not of that type on Hunter 5." Now he acknowledged that Collins's "most important motivation was science" and patient welfare was secondary. When asked what the study found, Goldenberg replied, "I don't know whether it was all worthwhile, frankly."[98] (His criticisms of Collins did not, however, extend to the procedure itself. In 1971, he recommended the operation for another patient in Wald's study. In a 1975 coauthored article, he praised new techniques for conducting a hypophysectomy and concluded that it was "still an integral part of therapy in selected patients" with metastatic breast cancer.[99])

Like Carson, Cohen was able to return home after the procedure, but she too did not survive very long. At the beginning of March, Goldenberg informed Cohen's husband that she had exhausted all possible treatment and they would "just have to continue to let her slip away."[100] A few days later, Cohen told the doctor she no longer felt safe or comfortable at home and asked him to readmit her to the hospital. She died there early on April 5, 1970.[101]

Conclusion

Wald hoped that she and Goldenberg could work together as equals, prefiguring the kind of relationships between nurses and doctors she considered central to the hospice ideal. Soon, however, she began to view him more as an impediment than as an ally. He opposed nonhierarchical arrangements in principle, resisted her attempts to reorder authority relationships between doctors and nurses, and declared he alone could determine his patients' best interests. Despite his avowed commitment to absolute honesty, an item at the forefront of Wald's agenda, he employed various strategies to keep bad news from them. Her condemnation of his practices of concealment had little impact.

Wald did, however, exert some influence on one issue. Her complaints about Collins's treatment of Cohen forced Goldenberg to confront the conflict between his roles as a physician and as an investigator. He was both a prominent researcher at a major academic medical center and an unusually compassionate breast cancer surgeon. He had joined Wald's study because he viewed hospital care for people approaching death as inhumane and fervently wanted to transform it. Nothing so sharply clashed with that goal as the use of dying patients as human subjects. By appealing to Goldenberg's empathetic side, Wald was gradually able to convince him that his colleagues had treated a dying woman callously, that research was not the same as therapy, and that investigators too often sacrificed patient needs in pursuit of scientific advancement.

3

Caring across Cultures

Wald became deeply engaged with all the patients and kin she studied, but two cases were especially important to her. They lasted the longest and involved some of the most complex personal issues and family relationships. Examining those cases enables us to perceive how she and other members of the research team understood their roles, the types of assistance they offered, the values that informed the study, and the ways patients and family members responded to the care they received. This chapter explores one of those cases; the following chapter discusses the other.

Wald first learned about Nunzio Rossi early in 1969 from his son Robert, who had arrived from southern Italy before the rest of the family and now owned a grocery store where Wald frequently shopped. A sixty-year-old construction worker, Nunzio had followed in 1960 with his wife, Allegra, and six other children. By February 6, 1969, when Wald decided to study the case, he had been sick for several months. Complaining of abdominal pain the previous summer, he had entered a community hospital close to his home. In November, his health had suddenly deteriorated, and he had been transferred to a ward at Yale New Haven Hospital (YNHH) for patients involved in research. There he underwent extensive bowel surgery. Because he had lost eight inches of bowel, he could consume nothing by mouth; instead, he received a mixture of coconut oil, wheat starch, and amino acids intravenously. A serious heart condition further complicated his recovery. Soon after Wald began to care for him, he fell into coma, emerging two days later but remaining seriously ill.

The case highlights the difficulty of studying an individual with an uncertain prognosis. Time after time, doctors predicted Nunzio's imminent demise, only to find they had erred. Convinced he should be considered a dying man, Wald insisted that his comfort be the top priority. But as he continued to survive, his doctors were able to justify their recommendations for aggressive treatment. The case also illustrates the problem of caring for patients and their relatives who spoke a different language and belonged to a culture that members of the research team viewed as inferior. Robert was the only family member fluent in English. The others had various levels of knowledge, but all felt more comfortable speaking Italian. Having traveled to Italy, Wald had acquired what she called "tourist Italian," which she acknowledged was far from adequate. None of the other health professionals and researchers claimed even that much. Although a translator occasionally was available, doctors and nurses repeatedly expressed uneasiness about caring for people with whom they communicated imperfectly or not at all. "How I *wish* I understood Italian!" Wald exclaimed at a moment of extreme frustration. She tried to learn the language but admitted progress was very slow.[1]

The language barrier led the doctors, nurses, social workers, and researchers involved in the case to rely on either ethnic stereotypes or personal experiences with Italian patients. Italian immigrants had a reputation for being overly "emotional."[2] Because Wald continually urged patients and their families to express their feelings, her repeated use of that term in reference to the Rossis needs some explanation. When she stressed the pejorative connotations of emotionality, she meant that people were too volatile, could not think rationally about critical issues, and were on the brink of collapse.

Soon after meeting the family, she announced that one of her primary goals was to resolve ongoing conflicts between Nunzio and Robert, enabling them to discuss mortality. A social worker involved in the case argued that her experience suggested that men "from that background" were unlikely to speak about illness and death. In response, Wald gave the example of a young Italian couple she had met at St. Christopher's in London. After the wife learned she was dying, she and her husband were able to communicate and "work together in the most beautiful way." Despite the many differences between the two cases, she intended to help the Rossi father and son collaborate equally well.[3]

Accounts of generational conflicts among Italian American families may help us understand their estrangement. Immigrant parents complained bitterly that their American-born children had abandoned traditional values and practices.[4] Although Robert was himself an immigrant, he must have seemed very foreign to Nunzio. Robert had lived much longer in the United States, spoke fluent English, was far better educated, and had climbed into the middle class. While Nunzio struggled to support his family with menial jobs, Robert had a successful store in Westport, the wealthy town where Wald lived. It is likely that Robert's rejection of family customs enraged his father, while Nunzio's expectation of obedience infuriated his son.

A deep fissure also existed between Robert and his siblings. Like their father, his brothers were all physical laborers. They resented the money that had been spent on his education. He was embarrassed by their work clothes and broken English. The most serious clash concerned modern medicine. As the head of the family during his father's illness, Robert had placed Nunzio in YNHH, a major academic medical center, over the objections of his mother and siblings. They had wanted Nunzio to enter St. Raphael's Hospital, a smaller, Catholic, and less research-oriented facility. And Nunzio's experience had done little to convince them of the superiority of modern medicine. Despite the many months he had spent in the hospital and the many therapies to which he had been subjected, he remained extremely ill. Now Robert demanded that the doctors transfer his father back to the research ward. The rest of the family insisted that Nunzio not be involved in any further studies and return home as soon as possible.

Wald initially sided with Robert, whom she knew best and considered "the most Americanized." The other children and their parents were "what we call in Westport, you know, kind of 'greasers,' day laborers, people who are interested in cars and [have] simple values." The father "didn't have any outside interests, just family." His was a "very, very restricted kind of life."[5] As she became better acquainted with the other family members, however, she changed her allegiance. Robert's open contempt for his siblings and parents offended her. And she began to view his trust in modern medicine as greatly exaggerated. Robert believed the doctors had the power to keep his father alive almost indefinitely and continually urged them to provide the most intensive therapy. Believing Nunzio was close to the end, she argued that the major goal should be to help him die well.

The most urgent issue was finding a place for him. As long as he was in the research ward, a grant had covered the cost of his care. Since moving to a general medical bed, however, he had been responsible for the fee. Hospital insurance plans had spread rapidly among all sectors of the population after World War II, and Nunzio was one of the many workers who had Blue Cross through his union. He could not, however, afford the deductible for long. He had saved enough money to buy a house but had nothing left over. During the six months he had been too sick to work, he and his wife had relied entirely on the earnings of the one son still living at home. Moreover, because his doctors were unsure whether he would die or recover soon, the hospital demanded his discharge. Since the early twentieth century, hospitals had tried to weed out chronic care patients. One reason was efficiency. During the months one such person might occupy a bed, the hospital could care for many people with acute diagnoses. In addition, medical attention focused increasingly on treatments for acute illnesses. Assuming that their graduates would interact solely with acute-care people, nursing and medical schools wanted to affiliate only with facilities filled with patients whose problems could be quickly as well as successfully resolved.[6] Thus although

Robert continually pressed the doctors to find a way to keep his father in the hospital, he could not prevail.

The hospital social worker responsible for finding an alternative bed quickly eliminated nursing homes from consideration. Nursing homes had arisen in the wake of the 1935 Social Security Act. Seeking to curtail the use of almshouses, the law stipulated that blind and needy people could receive aid only if they lived at home or in private institutions. During the next few decades, the number of facilities grew rapidly. The enactment of Medicare and Medicaid in 1965 imposed regulations to ensure that all nursing homes provided skilled nursing care. Two years later, a survey reported that a growing number of Connecticut facilities furnished nursing and therapeutic services.[7] Nevertheless, the social worker could find none in the area capable of changing Nunzio's IV. Chronic disease hospitals represented another possibility. Nunzio fit the profile of the typical patient at such a facility—elderly, low income, prior treatment in an acute care hospital, and with a severe, long-term health problem.[8] But most chronic disease hospitals, like many nursing homes, provided miserable care.[9] The social worker located three chronic disease hospitals for which Nunzio might be eligible before deciding they were "not very nice."[10]

The remaining option was to send Nunzio home. Although that was his preference and that of most of his family, the doctor and nurse responsible for his treatment feared he could not survive there for long. Health professionals and social workers had long asserted that families lacked the knowledge and skill needed to deliver adequate medical care at home; poor people were assumed to be especially unsuitable caregivers.[11] And Nunzio's case presented special difficulties. Ian M. Shenk, a gastroenterology fellow, noted that Nunzio's IV needed to be changed often, "sometimes in the middle of the night." That procedure had become so difficult that Shenk "had to spend a half an hour with it the other night." Although Wald promised to visit the house regularly, she did not believe she could handle the IV for a man with such poor veins. No one could imagine Nunzio's wife and children assuming that responsibility. Shenk also argued that because most family members were ignorant of the benefits Nunzio had received from his hospital stay, they would rely on more traditional methods of healing and feed him excessively. While Robert did value modern medicine, he had other faults and could not be trusted. Shenk had become enraged when Robert insisted on staying in the room during a delicate procedure in violation of hospital policy. Shenk was even more irate when Robert claimed to have enough medical knowledge to understand his father's physical problems. Shenk explained how he had tried to set Robert straight. After hearing the previous week that his father possibly had had a stroke, Robert "wanted to know if it was a stroke in the big brain or the little brain and I knew what he was talking about but I purposefully pretended that I didn't because I wanted him to realize how limited his scientific knowledge was so that he would not pretend to be such an expert; what he was trying to say was whether it was the cerebrum or the cerebellum."[12]

Nurse Blood, the head nurse in the research unit, expressed even greater contempt for the family. "A dying patient's family creates a chronic problem for nurses," wrote sociologists Barney G. Glaser and Anselm L. Strauss. "Family members are relatively easy to handle one at a time, but as a group they can join forces to put pressure on the nurse to give them better visiting hours, more information, special treatment, and so on. Nurses must control the family so as to keep disturbing scenes at a minimum."[13] But Blood had been unable to exert authority over Nunzio's relatives. Unlike "normal" families, they were constantly around, telling the doctors what to do and demanding special favors from the nurses.[14] Blood also noted that Nunzio was incontinent, a difficulty many families were reluctant to handle. When Shenk commented that they could just wait and see how the family coped with the father voiding in his bed, Blood angrily retorted, "Right. And stooling in the bed. Let them have it full blast." She too disliked Robert. She asserted that although he dressed better than his brothers, his modern clothes could not hide his imperfect acculturation; when under stress, he "reverted to his Italianese background."[15] Like Shenk, she had been especially irate when Robert had claimed medical competence. Believing he was qualified to handle the IV, he had made serious errors tampering with it. And she shared Shenk's fear that Allegra would try to heal her husband with her own cooking. Convinced that Allegra would refuse to comply with the instructions about his diet and reverse all the benefits he had received from his hospital care, Blood urged Shenk not to let him go home.

The possibility of Nunzio's discharge also worried Wald. Because she hoped to involve the Visiting Nurse Association in any home care plan, she met with the supervisor of a local agency. Pointing out the need for institutional care, the supervisor asked about the children: "Are they fairly stable or are they the excitable Italians where they under stress start . . ." Wald finished the question: "to fall apart" and then added that "it makes the whole business of taking him home and into their setting much more of a problem than it would be if the family were in better command of their emotions." The supervisor noted that the family's behavior was common among "this particular ethnic group."[16]

Despite the growing emphasis on patient autonomy, Shenk insisted that he alone had the authority to make the decision. But he had begun to waver. Observing Nunzio's suffering and the family conflicts it ignited, Shenk had decided that the patient's continued existence had little value to him or anyone else. By accelerating death, home care could end everyone's misery. Uncertain how to proceed, Shenk took the unusual step of consulting Nunzio and Allegra. Shenk made it clear that Nunzio would survive longer in the hospital, but Nunzio viewed the facility as a jail and his wife wanted to care for him at home. Pointing to the small statue of the Madonna they had placed on the windowsill, they stated that Nunzio's future was "now in the hands of God."[17] Although Robert A. Orsi's classic book *The Madonna of 115th Street: Faith and Community in Italian Harlem, 1880–1950* covers a different East Coast urban area and ends before the Rossis met with Shenk, it helps us understand their comment. According to Orsi, devotion to the Madonna had a central place in Southern Italian immigrant culture; numerous accounts circulated about her ability to heal sickness along with other major troubles.[18] With little evidence of the effectiveness of modern medicine, the couple must have been especially eager to place their trust in divine intervention.

Although delighted that the patient and his wife had participated in decision-making, Wald now confronted an enormous task. Convinced that Nunzio was on the verge of death, Shenk urged her to get him home as soon as possible. With "death breathing down on our necks," she rushed to make preparations. By February 17, the date of Nunzio's discharge, she announced she was ready. Shenk had prepared detailed instructions for the local doctor and visiting nurses. Although both Shenk and Wald had argued that only a physician could change Nunzio's IV, Blood had tried to teach the family how to perform that procedure. She also had "literally a drug store" to send home with the patient, including medications, food, blender, cases of IV fluids, and an IV stand.[19] Wald had located other supplies, met with Dr. Steinberg, who practiced in the community and would assume responsibility for the case, and made financial arrangements. Nunzio's insurance plan was one of the few that covered home care; because he needed skilled nursing care after a hospital stay, he met the restrictive criteria. As a result, Wald was able to hire three private-duty nurses to cover the twenty-four-hour day. She also applied for welfare on Nunzio's behalf to pay for equipment and medications.

Although Wald received various kinds of assistance from Shenk and Blood, she clearly had antagonized them. Their primary complaint was that she had not maintained proper professional distance, a criticism she would hear over and over. In this instance, the charge stemmed from the belief that Nunzio was not worth all the attention he had received. Blood argued that had Wald not been so emotionally engaged, he would have been discharged much earlier and "that would have been the end of it."[20] A 1964 article by Glaser and Strauss suggests that Blood again expressed widespread views. The nurses the sociologists studied bestowed the most care on patients with the highest "social value": "Extra 'good will' efforts are made to talk with them, to keep up their spirits, to make them comfortable, and to watch for sudden changes in their condition."[21] Characteristics that influenced social evaluations included age, class background, occupation, and education, all traits on which Nunzio would have scored poorly.

Wald reported that Nunzio's first days at home justified all the work involved in getting him there. He was "tremendously, tremendously pleased" to be out of the hospital. She undoubtedly was unaware of the condescension she displayed when she wrote that it was a "sweet little house," adding that "the backyard isn't anything great to look out on, but it's his." Although she previously had said he had no friends, his "cronies" came the day he arrived to toast his health.[22] But myriad problems immediately arose. While unpacking the medications with Wald, Robert became ill. That night Wald had to rush Nunzio to a local emergency room to get his IV fixed. Soon, a severe stomach virus spread through the entire household. And the family members quickly confirmed negative stereotypes of Italian immigrants. As Wald had predicted, the family seemed to have no emotional strength. Furious that his wishes had been disregarded, Robert stayed away from the house and offered little assistance. Fights erupted on his rare appearances. Another son refused to leave his bed after recovering from the flu. The wife of a third son went to live at her mother's house, protesting that he spent too much time with his father. One daughter worked full-time. And according to Wald, she was too "excitable" to be able to help even if she had been available.

Allegra especially seemed to conform to the stereotype of the volatile Italian. Because she was too tense to sleep, Wald concluded she must have been psychotic at one point. When Shenk protested that Wald did not know enough about either the family or Italian culture to make such a judgment, she agreed but continued to refer to Allegra as emotionally unstable. Nunzio's constant demands appeared to contribute to the pressure on his wife. If she seemed weaker at home than she had in the hospital, her husband suddenly was transformed from a frail, elderly patient into a man who could "tell everyone just what to do."[23] From the couch in the living room, he directed the snow plows outside. His wife and children feared him. His physical presence contributed to his commanding authority. Wald assumed that his military experience explained "his very straight bearing."[24] She too hesitated to challenge him, even when his actions violated her principles. Because she had anticipated that the Rossis would not accept an African American in the house, she was unsurprised when Nunzio complained that the night nurse, "a Negro" woman, "was scratching at herself all night long and that he didn't want her bugs to get over him and therefore he wanted to have her out of the house."[25] Wald may have been especially sensitive to this issue not only because she supported the civil rights movement but also because when she had attended the Yale University School of Nursing in the late 1940s, it had refused to admit African Americans.[26] Despite her respect for the nurse and disbelief that she had acted the way Nunzio described, Wald agreed to find a replacement.

She acted far more assertively when Nunzio was not involved. Undaunted by her limited Italian, she attempted to alleviate the fraught atmosphere. "I spend most of my time when I'm there reducing the tension," she reported. "When you go in you can feel the air—it's so hot and I just try to go around and see who's hottest and try to work with that person."[27] She demanded that the son lingering in bed get up and help care for his father. Hearing that she intended to reconcile the third son and his wife, Blood exclaimed, "You've become a marriage counselor, Mrs. Wald, along with everything else."[28] Later Wald was able to report that she had gotten the couple into a "more reasonable relationship."[29] Other tensions were not so easily diffused. Seven days after Nunzio arrived home, Wald noted that no one continued to enjoy his presence.

Financial problems added to the stress. Although Nunzio had qualified for welfare, the program delayed reimbursing suppliers and doctors, and the vendors began to demand payment. Moreover, because Shenk had assumed Nunzio could survive no more than three days at home, Wald had paid little attention to the likelihood that his coverage for nursing care would be quickly exhausted. But as the days passed and he remained alive, everyone began to worry. The only family member who could afford to pay out of pocket was Robert, but he had not wanted his father home and seemed unlikely to contribute.[30] Without visiting nurses, Allegra and her children would have to change the IV, a prospect that provoked profound anxiety among them. Wald previously had argued that the procedure was too complex for the family and only a highly qualified professional should perform it. Now, however, she attributed the family members' reluctance to assume that task to psychological vulnerability. "They're not gifted people by any stretch of the imagination," she wrote. The problem was that they could not accept "the emotional responsibility."[31]

In the end, a new health crisis forced the issue. Because Nunzio's IV was not changed for twenty hours, he developed a fever and returned to YNHH on February 28. Finding his father in a general medical bed, Robert insisted that the doctors transfer him back to the research ward, where an innovative therapy might be found to cure him. When they refused, Robert accused them of losing interest in his father because he no longer could participate in research. Wald agreed that the hospital viewed Nunzio primarily as an object of study, but she believed the doctors provided too much care rather than too little care. She argued that because he had undergone a rare surgery and survived longer than anyone had expected, he had become an interesting case. As a result, his doctors were conducting an experiment, "trying out various things without his permission."[32]

But there was little Wald could do. "My attempts to intrude myself in decision-making were jarring to the system," she later wrote.[33] No one wanted her opinion. The head nurse was uninterested in the "humanization part" of care.[34] The doctors allowed her to accompany them on their rounds one morning, but "at certain times I had to search for a spot where I could hear what they were saying and several times had to reposition myself when someone stepped in front of me and so closed me out of the inner circle."[35] When she tried to contribute to the discussion, the doctors turned their backs on her. A few days later "the doctors were right outside the room and the door was slightly ajar and I opened it a little bit so that I could listen and the doctor told me to shut the door."[36] For the first time, she acknowledged that intense involvement in a case might have a disadvantage. Her inability to influence decisions about Nunzio's care made her feel as "immobilized" as a patient, and she feared that her extreme frustration and anger had rendered her less competent as an observer.[37]

She was more successful forging a closer relationship with Allegra. Wald often drove her to and from the hospital, and as they rode together, Allegra steadily grew in Wald's estimation. Allegra was doing "a magnificent piece of work," Wald wrote. Allegra sometimes concentrated on her rosary, but often she talked. "Through the language difficulties," she freely expressed her sadness and anxiety. Wald also was impressed that she displayed the appropriate affect in the hospital.[38] No matter how depressed she felt, she looked cheerful when she entered Nunzio's room. With Wald's encouragement, she learned how to bathe him. When the doctors decided he could begin to have a more regular diet, she prepared *zambaione*, a custard containing eggs, Marsala, and sugar, one of the few dishes he was permitted to eat.[39]

As Nunzio's fever declined and he continued to defy predictions about an imminent death, the hospital again insisted he leave. Because home was no longer was an option, the social worker searched for alternatives. For the second time, Wald complained about her powerlessness. She wanted Nunzio to go to a nearby facility so Allegra could see him regularly. But hospitals traditionally had placed a low priority on the ability of poor families to visit patients, and the YNHH social worker seemed unconcerned that all the places she was considering were inaccessible by public transportation.[40] Wald was thus relieved when Nunzio was transferred to a hospital close to his home on April 28. Because Nunzio had stayed there the previous summer, it was very familiar to the entire family.

Proximity, however, could not forestall new tensions. Although the records do not indicate the source of the problems, they reveal that Allegra sometimes refused to visit. On those occasions, Nunzio became desperate, refusing to eat anything but the food she brought. Wald thus decided she had to help them complete the "piece of work" that "would make him feel that he's leaving his wife okay and [enable] her to say that I'm okay." Once again other researchers and health professionals challenged her presumption, arguing that Wald knew so little about the marital relationship and had such an imperfect grasp of Italian that it would be inappropriate for her to intervene in any way. Dr. Steinberg noted that the couple might be doing the best they could under the circumstances. And indeed, Allegra was far from "okay." Not only was she losing her husband, but her future looked extremely bleak. Although Robert was the oldest and wealthiest son, no one wanted him to be head of the household after his father's death. Without his money, Allegra would have to relinquish the house and live with one of her children. Wald, however, insisted it was her job to "try to bring [the couple] together and hold them together." Nunzio could die well only if she helped him complete all of his "unfinished business."[41] There is no indication that she fulfilled that goal.

Nor could she resolve the conflict between Robert and Nunzio. Despite her desire to facilitate better communication, the two men seemed more estranged than ever. On the few occasions Robert came to the hospital, he remained in the hall outside his father's room, talking to the staff. Wald's one attempt to intervene in their relationship backfired. Visiting Nunzio one day, she found him "infuriated at Robert and after a heated discussion in Italian on the phone banged the phone down." She explained what happened next: "I picked the receiver up again and said to Robert not to get angry. I was trying to protect Robert from his father's rage but even as I did it I realized this might make Mr. R. angry at me. Apparently it had."[42] The following day Nunzio announced he was "sick" of Wald and the doctors and wanted to be left alone. (Although she acknowledged feeling "crushed," Wald decided to continue delivering care; Nunzio appeared subdued for a few days but gradually resumed his previous mien.)[43] Robert was no more appreciative.

Although few reports from the next three months survive, Nunzio continued to stave off death. Despite the many troubles that had occurred when he had been home the previous February, he returned there on July 7. The records resume in the middle of the month, when the Rossis faced another critical decision. Several family members wanted Nunzio to visit relatives in Italy. Robert supported Dr. Steinberg, the local doctor, who urged Nunzio to enroll in George Washington Hospital in Washington, DC, where he could undergo a procedure unavailable in New Haven. Wald was leery of siding with one side over the other and incredulous that either plan was under consideration. It seemed preposterous for such a gravely ill man to travel abroad. But it was even more absurd for him to take a train to Washington, enter a new hospital, and be subjected to one more intervention. Wald accused Steinberg of subordinating the patient's needs to his own interests (presumably to learn more about the recommended procedure). And once again, she complained bitterly about being excluded from the decision-making process. Unable to make either Robert or Steinberg heed her advice, she felt "quite helpless and irritated."[44]

Nunzio, Allegra, and Robert departed for Washington on August 2. The trip was a disaster. Because they arrived in the rain, they had difficulty finding a taxi. The hospital claimed not to have known Nunzio was arriving, and he had to wait four hours for admission. That night he began vomiting and had chills. He died a few days later, after two massive heart attacks.

After hearing about Nunzio's death, Wald rushed to the house: "Mrs. Rossi threw her arms around me and was for a long time half crying, half speaking Italian. I just held her, and after about 15 minutes she calmed down."[45] Wald also had an important job to do. Her son Joel recalled that when Nunzio died, "he of course had lost a tremendous amount of body mass. My mother asked me if he could be buried in my Bar Mitzvah suit. I immediately said 'Yes.'"[46] She also visited the family at the funeral home and then attended the service.

Wald frequently noted the importance of continuing relationships with bereaved family members. Allegra especially seemed to welcome her ongoing involvement. The notes contain references to a visit Allegra made to the Walds' house in late September and a trip Wald made to the state welfare office with Allegra in early October. Although the welfare worker seemed pleasant enough, she also seemed "to have a tremendous lack of knowledge." Wald wondered what would happen to a family that did not have someone along like herself to question "the procedures and rulings."[47] When Wald phoned the house in late November, Allegra "answered and before I could even tell her who it was, she responded with a very warm, 'Oh Mrs. Wald' and I was amazed at how much we could speak together."[48] Early in March 1970, Allegra's granddaughter called to ask Wald to visit to discuss ongoing problems with the welfare office. She soon arrived, bringing flowers from her garden. When Allegra came down the stairs, "we embraced, kissing each other on both cheeks and as she took me in her arms she broke out into sobs." Allegra then told Wald the family news. Her own situation was much better than she had anticipated. She shared her house with her youngest son, who was now engaged. The couple planned to live on the top floor after their marriage, leaving the bottom one for her and covering much of the expense. Having failed to establish himself as the head of the family, Robert was now completely alienated. Neither Allegra nor any of her other children saw him. He also had distanced himself from Wald. Although she continued to shop at his store, he refused to acknowledge her presence.[49] But her relationship with other family members pleased her. She was thrilled to be invited to the youngest son's wedding. Occurring at the end of August, a year after Nunzio's death, it marked the end of the bereavement period. Wald's last notes about the Rossis includes a detailed description of the event.

Conclusion

Unable to communicate easily with most members of the Rossi family, health professionals and researchers viewed them in terms of stereotypes of Italian immigrants. Although Wald later would stress the importance of learning about the cultural practices of patients and kin, she appears to have been even more willing than most of her colleagues to proceed on the basis of imperfect information. On various occasions, other researchers protested that she was too unfamiliar with the Rossi family life to follow the course she had chosen. But by the time the case closed, she could point to several major accomplishments. Undertaking complex logistical duties, she had enabled Nunzio to spend ten precious days at home with his family. She had ensured that he was not sent to a facility too far for his wife to visit. She had interceded between the family and the complex welfare bureaucracy. And although initially wary of Allegra, Wald eventually established a warm and supportive relationship with her. What she could not do was promote the family harmony she considered the precondition for a good death. Despite her best efforts, deep cleavages continued to divide the Rossi family.

Medical care was the most highly charged issue. Although the records tell little about the Rossi family's health beliefs, most family members were far less willing than Robert to embrace modern medicine. Nunzio's long hospital stay must have done little to change their minds. We can only imagine how alien and intimidating YNHH must have seemed to people who had little command of English and whom doctors and nurses treated with disdain. And despite the massive technology the facility contained, it had failed to restore Nunzio to health.

Robert's views brought him into conflict with the hospital staff as well as with his family. He demanded far more from modern medicine than it possibly could deliver. Convinced that the next treatment could save his father, he continually pressed the staff to try one more intervention. Wald had the opposite complaint. She asserted that the hospital's focus on prolonging life compelled Nunzio's doctors to subject him to many useless treatments. Even worse, she argued, they had continued to view him as an object of inquiry even after he left the research ward. She charged that physicians were experimenting on him and suspected that his local doctor had recommended the trip to Washington, DC, to learn about a procedure administered there. Her inability to change hospital culture bolstered her resolve to found a facility for dying people that was entirely separate from the established health care system. When she had tried to convert Nunzio's doctors to her way of thinking about terminal care, they had shunned her completely.

4

Hope, Blame, and Acceptance

As the Rossi case progressed, Wald and her colleagues discussed what kind of patient they wanted to study next. Wald argued that she had put ten times as much effort into working with the Rossis as would have been required for an English-speaking family; she was determined not to have to struggle with a language barrier again. Others noted the importance of studying a patient with an illness like cancer, which typically followed a predictable trajectory. Because Nunzio had repeatedly outlived projections, it had been difficult to determine at what point he should be considered dying. The second major case fulfilled both criteria.

By November 1969, when that case opened, Wald had begun to select study participants solely from Goldenberg's roster of breast cancer patients. The ones she chose were women he believed had a three-month life expectancy. All had received their diagnoses in either the 1950s or—more commonly—the 1960s. During those decades, the reigning medical approach to breast cancer had two facets: early discovery of disease and radical surgery. Since its creation in 1913, the American Society for the Control of Cancer (later renamed the American Cancer Society) had tried to counter the fatalism surrounding the disease. Arguing that a breast cancer diagnosis was not a death sentence, the organization encouraged women to find breast lumps as soon as possible. By World War II, a massive health-education campaign had developed in the United States, promising that breast cancer would neither kill nor maim any woman who remained vigilant, regularly examined her breasts, and reported all suspicious signs to her doctor.[1]

The early detection movement rested on a belief that the dominant treatment could cure breast cancer in its initial stages. Most doctors followed Johns Hopkins University surgeon William Stewart Halsted, who pioneered radical mastectomies. That operation had devastating consequences, causing serious chest deformities, including hollow areas under the collarbones and armpits, and, in some cases, lymphedema (arm or hand swelling), pain, and mobility problems. In the early 1970s, Goldenberg joined a growing chorus of surgeons who argued that breast cancer was a systemic rather than a local disease and that radical mastectomies were no more effective than less aggressive procedures.[2] By the end of the decade, a combination of accumulating scientific evidence, patient dissatisfaction, and women's health activism convinced the majority of surgeons to abandon the Halsted mastectomy. But as late as 1968, the year before Wald inaugurated her study, the great majority of women diagnosed with breast cancer underwent that operation.[3]

Although the feminist breast cancer movement did not emerge until the 1970s, earlier generations of patients were not entirely passive. In a 1954 magazine article titled "I Had Breast Cancer," Terese Lasser declared, "A deplorable curtain of silence hangs about this subject and it is time we lift it."[4] Patients often failed to disclose their diagnoses, even to intimates, and doctors routinely listed other causes on death certificates. Lasser attempted to pierce that silence by founding Reach to Recovery. Long before the establishment of support groups for people confronting various afflictions, Reach to Recovery organized breast cancer survivors. Visiting other women immediately after diagnosis or surgery, volunteers discussed the aftereffects of radical mastectomies, explained how women could regain mobility in their arms, and provided fashion advice. Like advocates of both early detection and Halsted mastectomies, Reach to Recovery emphasized hope and optimism. The organization's literature preached that prostheses could not only create a normal appearance but also facilitate healing and that any woman with sufficient willpower could rapidly return to health.[5] By 1969, when Reach to Recovery became part of the American Cancer Society, it had grown into a massive organization, serving thousands of newly diagnosed women.[6]

The flip side of glorifying cure was denigrating those who either died or were seriously ill. Members of the second group were held responsible for their own misfortunes. Doctors who previously might have viewed advanced disease as inevitable or the result of their own incompetence could blame patients for having failed to recognize the first signs of cancer and take corrective action. A 1945 drug advertisement that appeared in numerous popular magazines contrasted "wise" and "foolish" women with breast cancer. The "wise" woman had quickly reported her breast lump to her doctor; as a result, she had no complications from surgery and "recovered completely." The accompanying photograph depicted a healthy, smiling woman at home with her two children. Because the "foolish" woman had delayed bringing her lump to a physician's attention, the disease had spread so widely that a mastectomy could not help. She was shown dying in a hospital room with a nurse but no family.[7]

Although we cannot know to what extent the women Wald studied had absorbed the message of personal responsibility, the belief that they had brought their fate upon themselves must have intensified the suffering of many. The emphasis on normal appearance imposed special burdens. The many films and posters of the cancer awareness movement never showed the physical realities of the end of life.[8] Even the "foolish" woman in the drug company advertisement was pictured with a round face and a full head of hair, a blanket tactfully covering the rest of her body. Breast cancer patients who were close to death had to hide not only the loss of a breast but also symptoms commonly viewed as abhorrent. Many participants in Wald's study had large ulcerated tumors that caused intense shame. Clothes could conceal them from sight but failed to mask their odor.

The ideology of the major cancer organizations also clashed with Wald's mission. Those groups tried to engender a new openness about breast cancer without challenging the traditional evasion of mortality. Wald wanted the people under her care to stare unflinchingly at death and summon the emotional and spiritual resources needed to confront it. With Marion Weber, the patient in the second case, she achieved only limited success. After meeting Marion in Goldenberg's breast cancer clinic in fall 1969, Wald realized they had much in common. They were at the same stage of life, had children the same ages, and belonged to the same culture. Wald also quickly understood that Marion's situation was especially tragic. Born in 1925, she had been living with breast cancer for ten years. Despite a radical mastectomy, the disease had continued to progress and was now very advanced. Her husband had died five years earlier after struggling with the effects of a brain injury for a decade. Previously a school teacher, Marion had taken leave from her job many weeks before meeting Wald and seemed unlikely to ever return. She had sole responsibility for three daughters who were still dealing with their father's long period of disability and death and now had to witness their mother's rapid deterioration. The oldest was Susanna (seventeen). The two younger ones had their own serious problems. Helen (fifteen) was deaf in one ear. Rose (thirteen) was emotionally fragile.

Marion must have felt profoundly isolated with her troubles. Several months earlier, she had moved her family from New York City to be near her mother (referred to as "Mrs. Klein" in the notes) and her sister, Alice Hirsch, in the New Haven area. But she and her mother had long been emotionally estranged. Although Marion was much closer to her sister, Alice had her own family and was often unavailable. Moreover, she and her husband departed for a Florida vacation in January 1970 and then repeatedly postponed their return. Once back home, she became preoccupied with planning a fund-raising luncheon for a major charity. As a newcomer in her community, Marion was without the friends and neighbors who might have rallied around her. Nor could she share her experience with fellow sufferers. Very sick patients interacted rarely, if ever, in Goldenberg's waiting room. And although Reach to Recovery tried to create a sense of community among breast cancer survivors, it had little to offer a woman whose health was steadily worsening.[9]

Three other issues demanded immediate attention. Marion seemed unaware she was dying. Goldenberg acknowledged that his reluctance to reveal grim prognoses might have contributed to the problem. When he knew the disease had spread to Marion's lungs, he assured her she had nothing more serious than a cold. When Wald argued that patients deserved honesty, Goldenberg explained that Marion "was using the mechanism of denial, and probably needed to do this."[10] By the end of December 1970, however, he agreed that she should make practical and emotional preparations and promised to tell her the truth at her next clinic visit. It was soon clear he had failed. Although she must have known experientially that she would not recover, several weeks would elapse before she would admit how gravely ill she was.

The next two problems stemmed from the first. Because death could occur at any time, it was imperative that Marion's daughters understand her condition. The two older girls intuitively grasped it although no one had explicitly told them their mother was approaching the end. The youngest girl, however, continued to believe she could be cured. Convinced that Marion suffered from pleurisy or another nonfatal disease, Rose asked Wald if she would come to the celebratory dinner she planned to hold. Rose also urged her mother to go back to work, eat more to gain weight, and even marry again because she had been healthier before her husband died. Horrified by the idea of the girls finding their mother dead one morning, Wald wanted her to prepare them. "Wouldn't Marion feel better as she is dying to know that the kids have come to peace with this and can master it?" Wald asked her colleagues. "This would be marvelous information for her to have, that these kids went around and did all that problem solving. I would be thrilled if I knew my kids were doing it."[11] Marion apparently felt differently.

The precariousness of Marion's health also made plans for the girls' futures an immediate concern. Wald was especially insistent that Marion had an obligation to make arrangements, and she repeatedly pressed Marion not to leave that job undone. As she wrote in another case, "I feel so strongly that the patient has a responsibility to the family members, or all those other important people who are around them."[12] Nevertheless, Marion continually evaded the subject. One researcher speculated that she was loath to bring new sorrow to her daughters, who had endured so much tragedy, by discussing what would happen after her death. Another suggested that Marion feared that discussing what would happen after her death would make it seem more real.

The most compelling explanation may be that no good option existed. Both Goldenberg and Wessel, the other doctor on the research team, were convinced that "when the chips were down," their colleague Dr. Gordon Harris would take the girls. He was a local pediatrician as well as Marion's cousin. But he soon made it clear that he had no intention of doing so. In the middle of March, the girls said they had not seen him since before Christmas. In other cases, Wald and her colleagues had urged family members to provide more care to dying patients; Harris, however, received a pass from Wessel, who argued that Harris had lived with Marion's family for ten years while growing up and thus was much closer than an ordinary cousin. Because he was "so caught up in this crisis with his own feelings," it would be inappropriate to push him to assume responsibility. Harris paid for some medical supplies and participated in a few family conferences about the girls, but in other ways, he kept his distance.[13]

Although Mrs. Klein was able to prepare evening meals, she too was ill and could do little more. Moreover, as Goldenberg explained, "Marion's mother drives her to complete distraction to the point where she really gets physically upset about this woman and her constant nagging of the kids when they are home, and her great compulsions about how the house should be cleaned."[14] Klein complained that no one appreciated all the work she did. Both Goldenberg and Wald urged her to spend less time at the house.

Alice might have seemed the most obvious guardian, but Marion's daughters refused to consider her. When Marion and her children first arrived from New York, they had lived with the Hirsches, but the cousins had not gotten along. Alice's husband Mort freely acknowledged that he "could not stand" his nieces, and the two sisters had very different parenting styles. The girls' father had been the authority figure in the household, and since his death, they had enjoyed their mother's greater leniency. Alice, by contrast, demanded proper manners and strict obedience. The Hirsches also were considerably wealthier. As Wald noted, the family belonged to a "fashionable set" in Hamden, a town north of New Haven. After leaving the Hirsch house, Marion and her daughters moved to an apartment in a low-income area in the city. Although information about Marion's income after she stopped working is lacking, we know she had difficulty making ends meet. As in the Rossi case, Wald made her sympathies clear. She had described Ruth Cohen, the affluent woman who underwent a hypophysectomy, as leading a "superficial" life and now directed the same charge at the Hirsches. With their quick intelligence and lively curiosity, the three Weber girls could not fit into the Hirsches' "superficial country-club" household.

Although Wald struggled to establish a personal connection to Marion, Goldenberg immediately formed a warm relationship with her. His bond with her oldest daughter was even closer. In the fall of 1969, Susanna made an appointment to discuss her mother's condition and afterwards visited and called often. Goldenberg soon felt a strong sense of responsibility for the girl. After one meeting, Goldenberg berated himself when he realized he had neglected to ask Susanna about her college plans. Goldenberg did, however, find a therapist for her at the Connecticut Mental Health Center and offered to discuss her failing Spanish grade with the high school principal. He also dispensed advice. When Susanna said that she planned to go on a ski trip over the school vacation to escape the tension that drove her "crazy" at home, Goldenberg reminded her of her obligation to her mother and urged her to ask Marion if she could manage without her for a week.[15] Although Susanna made it clear that she derived comfort from those conversations,

Goldenberg was more ambivalent. Unlike Wald, he did not seek intimate relationships with relatives and thus insisted that this case not set a precedent. With responsibility for more than three hundred patients a year, he vowed to never again get so involved with a family member.[16]

Wald's initial attempts to care for Marion met rebuff. Because Marion had a large lesion that she admitted "just disgusted her," Wald continually offered to help manage it. By the 1960s most people believed that only trained nurses had the expertise to clean and dress wounds from advanced cancer. Marion, however, insisted that she could care for hers alone. Wald was thus pleased when Marion asked if she could address Wald by her first name. "I felt she had made a move toward me," Wald commented.[17] Soon afterwards, Marion invited her home to administer Vitamin B12 shots, which she believed had given her husband added energy close to his death.

Wald arrived for her first visit on February 25, 1970. After giving the injection, she was allowed to dress the chest lesion, which she agreed was horrendous. Marion was very weak, "huffing and puffing" just walking around the room. Wald also met Mrs. Klein and two of the girls. Although pleased to observe Marion's easy relationship with her daughters, Wald found the youngest girl's behavior disturbing. "A bright, chubby" girl, Rose was anxious, "taking everything in and punching the pillows as she talked."[18]

Leaving the house, Wald made a comment indicating that she was Jewish. Mrs. Klein's eyes lit up when she realized that the woman offering her services shared many of the same values and attitudes. And Wald undoubtedly was relieved to discover she could draw on her cultural heritage as she tried to deal with the myriad problems confronting the household. Rose was not the only concern. Walking to her car, Wald "had the feeling of four people screaming out loud for help."[19] That evening she found it difficult to "disentangle myself from them in thought." She accompanied her husband to a concert but could not concentrate and "gave into an urge" to phone the girls' uncle at the intermission.[20]

As a woman who was intent on controlling her own life, Wald respected Marion's determination to manage hers as long as possible. When Goldenberg asked how Marion felt about letting her sister and mother help with the housework, she angrily replied, "I just don't like to be waited on, that's all, but I have to be."[21] In early March, Wald met Marion at the hospital door while her while her daughter parked the car. "Because Marion swayed slightly," Wald wrote, "I said you don't want a wheelchair do you? And she said, wheelchair, of course not! And I said, Oh, don't bite my head off." Wald then commented that she would have felt the same way.[22] Wald thus was not surprised that when she returned to dress the wound and administer injections, Marion refused other types of assistance. Deteriorating health, however, soon forced her to reconsider. Wald's reports traced Marion's decline. At the end of February, she weighed less than a hundred pounds and had "great shortness of breath and a lot of difficulty getting around."[23] In the middle of March, she seemed "agitated at the slightest thing" and could do little more than sit in her chair at home.[24] Wald wondered how long she could remain there. At the end of the month, she was just barely holding her own. In early April, she seemed to be fading away. The odor of the wound permeated the house; she could not sit at the dinner table for more than fifteen minutes and had great difficulty climbing the stairs at night.

When Wald began visiting every day, Alice thanked her for rendering the intimate physical care she would have found repellent. Alice may have been less pleased as Wald gradually inserted herself into the household by taking over the nonmedical tasks that became too onerous for Marion. As Wald folded the laundry, cooked dinners, washed dishes, and helped the girls with homework and picked them up from school, she viewed herself as sustaining rather than undermining Marion's independence. "Marion is trying desperately to keep in control," Wald commented, "and I am trying very hard to keep her that way."[25] Wald also solicited practical and financial assistance from local agencies. As she had discovered when caring for Nunzio Rossi, very little was available. Marion's greatest need was for a homemaker to help in the early evening, when the household became especially chaotic. But such assistance was expensive and virtually impossible to find.

Above all, Wald provided the companionship Marion craved. Wald usually stayed through the early evening, sharing a drink and chatting with Marion until dinner was ready. Some days Wald drove her through the countryside for pleasure or downtown to run errands. On at least one occasion, they went out for ice cream. Their conversations often focused on Marion's daughters. When Marion worried that they would be underfoot during a week-long school holiday, Wald recommended activities for each. She also supported Marion in her interactions with the girls. When Marion told Rose she could not go out in the clothes she was wearing, Wald made her go upstairs and change. When her suggestions for her mother's recovery began to irritate Marion, Wald took Rose out of the house and made her promise to keep her feelings to herself when Wald was not around. Because Marion complained that Susanna was often away, Wald implored her to spend more time at home to manage her sisters and help with her mother's care. And when Marion finally indicated that she knew she was dying, Wald tried to help her prepare emotionally. Wald encouraged her to express her feelings of grief, anger, and fear; promised to remain with her to the end; and reassured her that all three children were strong enough to cope with her death.

Wald tried to understand and attend to the emotional needs of other family members as well. She sympathized with Mrs. Klein's troubles and tried to mediate between her and the rest of the family. Rose remained the primary worry, and Wald continued to seek opportunities to be alone with her. When she began to irritate her mother, Wald took her on errands. "We had a chance to talk a bit," Wald wrote after a trip to the grocery store, "and I cautioned her that one of the things that she and I were going to have to be careful was not to baby her mother too much, that she really didn't seem to want it, and that we just would have to restrain ourselves, as it didn't seem to help. She was wonderful about it and said, yes, she knew and she understood but she wanted so much to help her." Wald also tried to allay Rose's worst fears. "She said if anything happens to her mother, I'll be ruined. I said Rosie, you're much too strong to be ruined, if anything happens, you're going to hurt a lot but you're not going to be ruined."[26]

As Wald became more and more engaged with the Weber family, she pushed professional boundaries still further by beginning to involve members of her own household. At one point, she suggested taking in Helen and Rose if no good option appeared before their mother died. Although she quickly abandoned that idea, she frequently bought Rose home for weekends. There she helped Wald with the cooking and her husband with outside work. Wald introduced Susanna to her daughter, Shari, who was close to her in age, and the two began to make their own plans to get together. Wald also melded the two households when she exchanged food between them, brought her dogs to entertain the younger girls, and invited all the Webers to her family seder.

Wald's lack of professional distance was thus even more extreme than it had been in the previous case. It also provoked much harsher criticism. Goldenberg was aghast when she mentioned the possibility of taking care of the girls after their mother died. "Oh, Florence," he exclaimed, "now you've really gone too far."[27] Although Wald usually could count on Wessel's support, he took advantage of her absence at a research meeting to confess that he was "a little bit heartsick" about her attachment to the girls. Her excessive devotion to their needs was "pathetic."[28] Both a Catholic priest and a social worker who met occasionally with the research team asserted that Wald had become too emotionally entangled in the case to be able to think clearly about the family's needs. And some members of the team wondered how much they could learn from such an atypical case. No other family confronting death could receive the same level of free services Wald provided.

Wald occasionally admitted that her commitment to the Webers imposed a cost on her as well, exhausting her physically and reducing the attention she could give her own family. When dinner time at the Weber house was especially hectic, she felt pulled in all directions and had trouble maintaining her equilibrium. At night she woke up worrying about the entire household. But her colleagues' criticisms of her emotional involvement infuriated her, and she staunchly defended her actions. One way was by reminding them that the primary goal of the study was to understand the needs of dying people and their families. Her mentor Peplau had asserted that "when immediate needs are met, more mature needs arise."[29] Wald insisted that only by satisfying the needs the Weber family presented could she possibly discern those beneath the surface.

Wald also pointed out that her greatest gratification derived from the close relationships she forged with Marion and her family, even though no one was as forthcoming as she wanted. Although Marion confessed her worries about her daughters, she refused to admit to her fears about her premature death. "There is a certain amount of frustration and anger that I'm picking up from Marion," Wald wrote after a terrifying new symptom emerged. "I've tried to share my feelings with her saying that it seems to me that she was irritable or angry," but "she denied it and said she wasn't aware of it."[30] Helen was especially uncommunicative, often remaining in another room watching television when Wald visited. When Wald asked direct questions, Helen either said little or just shrugged. Despite Wald's pleas, Susanna continued to find excuses to stay away from home. Nevertheless, Wald often reported the warmth of the greeting she received from the entire family. Rose sought her company whenever she visited, never hesitated to accompany her on errands, and seemed to enjoy weekends at her house. It is likely that Wald also found satisfaction in feeling indispensable. When she went on a short vacation on Long Island, she left her phone number and made the family promise to call immediately if death seemed imminent. She would fly back because no one else could provide her kind of care.

Wald had a new challenge on April 15, the date of the charity luncheon that had absorbed Alice's time and energy for several months. Wald assumed Marion was much too ill to attend, but Alice wanted her to go, and Goldenberg gave his consent. Wald helped her get ready and accompanied her to the affair. There Wald sharpened her disapproval of Alice and her husband. When

Mort Hirsch arrived, Wald was "rather taken aback with his brusqueness with Marion and his lack of warmth. It sort of chilled me to the bone." The wealth on display also alienated her. The country club was "opulent" and the large dining room "filled with beautifully coiffured women in elegant dresses." Wald felt "critical and angry" when she contrasted the "people who seemed to be wallowing in luxury" with Marion, "struggling valiantly against terrible odds."[31] The implication was that Alice was as insensitive toward Marion as her husband had been and both would be inappropriate guardians of their nieces.

Marion's daughters delighted in seeing her dressed up, but their happiness was fleeting. On April 18, they told Goldenberg that their mother was very confused. A few days later, they reported that her speech had become garbled. Fearing the disease had spread to her brain, Goldenberg admitted her to the hospital. There Wald saw how much Marion had come to rely on her support. When other people were around, Marion tried to suppress her emotions. Alone with Wald, however, she poured out her grief. One evening she began to weep uncontrollably. "I just held her in my arms," Wald wrote, "and rocked her back and forth." She later remarked that when emotionally involved in a case, she found "it helpful to the patient if tears well up in my eyes, not to hide them, to openly make the patient feel that they are not alone."[32] Now she reported that she was able to share Marion's sorrow. "I was crying too," she wrote.[33] Another sign of her deep involvement was less pleasing. She reported strange physiological symptoms, a pain at the base of her neck, failure to recover from laryngitis, and most alarmingly, "the same difficulty findings words that Marion had."[34]

As Marion's speech gradually improved, money worries became more prominent. Because she could not easily afford the hospital fee of seventy-five dollars a day, Goldenberg and Wald began to make plans to transfer her to a private home in Woodbridge that accepted people who needed assistance with routine activities. The daily rate was between fifteen and twenty dollars, depending on an individual's resources. The enterprise belonged to the category that Bruce C. Vladeck defined as "mom and pop" nursing homes:

"Typically, a woman, sometimes with nursing or similar training, would provide 'nursing home' services within her own residence." Most facilities "provided for no more than a handful of residents (a big nursing home was one with more than a dozen beds) and were staffed by the immediate family of the operator."[35] In this case, the owner was Lucia Hawkins, who lived there with her husband. A hospital social worker and a patient care coordinator described the residence as a "lovely home in an idyllic setting." They recommended it as "an excellent, restful, and pleasant atmosphere" for an "individual accustomed to 'gracious living.'" Although Hawkins was a licensed practical nurse and had an "excellent background in geriatrics and public health," she provided meals and other housekeeping services but no nursing care.[36] Goldenberg would often complain about the absence of nursing services, but Marion was relieved to be able to consider herself a boarder rather than a patient. She also was happy to learn that the home bore no resemblance to the various institutions her husband had entered during his long illness. At some, she noted, he had been totally neglected.

Nevertheless, when she realized she could not go home, she again fell into despair and began to sob. Although Wald reminded her that the previous day she had said she could accept that she might stay the same, get better, or get worse, she wailed, "Oh, but with a little bit of luck, a little bit of luck, I thought I could make it." When words provided little consolation, Wald again offered physical comfort. Marion "held out her two hands to me, and I held them, and I kissed her head and held her head between my hands and rocked her back and forth and then she began to become more composed."[37] Marion's hysterical weeping embarrassed Wald. Several months later, however, she viewed both incidents in a new light. Marion's behavior may have been out of place in a hospital, but it had been appropriate "in the sense of accepting and expressing what one feels about leaving life." Although Wald had condemned Allegra Rossi's emotional outbursts, she was glad Marion had felt free to "fall apart as much as she did."[38]

Klaus, who recently had joined the research team, had yet another response. Since the early twentieth century, nurses had employed various strategies to maintain self-control in the face of impending death. They also had sought to insulate themselves from the suffering they witnessed by cultivating detachment.[39] Although Klaus shared Wald's emphasis on empathy, she tried to remain less emotionally involved. While dressing Marion's wound, Klaus "looked up and she had this big tear coming from her eyes. She had very little expression on her face and I ignored the tear and continued the dressing. The lesion is so bad, I don't think I could bear her tears just then, or I would cry and be too upset to finish the dressing. So it just wasn't mentioned."

"Getting out of the hospital always seemed like a rebirth," wrote sociologist Arthur W. Frank about his own illness experience. "Hospitals deprive the senses," he explained. Once outside, he "was aware of real air and colors and textures."[40] Marion had a similar sense of renewal when she was finally discharged on May 8. Riding to the nursing home, she "seemed delighted and was marveling at how pretty everything looked."[41] Three days later, she "just seemed to be thoroughly relaxed in this beautiful home."[42] She reveled in the nature she could see from her room. When she felt well enough, she sat outside in the garden or on the porch.

Marion's growing disengagement from her daughters undoubtedly both derived from and reinforced her sense of serenity. Soon after arriving at the Hawkinses' house, she announced she would be happy to not see them every other day. After Wald brought Rose to the home one afternoon, she realized Marion experienced the visit as more an imposition than a pleasure.[43] When Helen called to ask whether she should get a haircut, Marion stated that she did not want to be bothered with such questions.[44] She also continued to distance herself from a far more serious matter. Concerns about the girls' futures suddenly had acquired a new urgency. The extant records do not reveal all the issues involved and who was responsible for making the decision, but the evidence indicates that the question had become extremely contentious. The researchers' proposal to find a young couple to live with the girls in their own house appealed to them but not all their relatives.

Although aware of the controversy swirling around her daughters, Marion indicated that she had no desire to get involved.

Wald and her colleagues struggled to make sense of Marion's behavior. Since the appearance of Kübler-Ross's *On Death and Dying* in November 1969, the research team had tried to apply her theory about the stages of grief. According to her schema, patients who had worked through their feelings of denial, anger, bargaining, and depression finally reached the zenith, acceptance. Although she emphasized the role of religion in helping people achieve acceptance, she insisted that faith was not a prerequisite. Any patient who "is allowed to grieve," whose "life is not artificially prolonged," and whose "family has learned to 'let go,' . . . will be able to die with peace and in a state of acceptance."

Acceptance thus clearly was essential to the growth process Wald and her colleagues sought to engender. But what exactly was it, and how could the researchers recognize it when they saw it? "Acceptance should not be mistaken for a happy stage," Kübler-Ross argued. Rather, "it is almost void of feelings. . . . While the dying person has found some peace and acceptance, his circle of interest diminishes. He wishes to be left alone or at least not stirred up by news and problems of the outside world."[45] With that definition in mind, Wald declared that Marion had attained acceptance. But then she reconsidered. Marion certainly seemed serene and withdrawn, but she had "unfinished business." In the previous case, Wald had used that term to refer to the emotional work the patient and his wife had to do to repair their relationship. Here Wald was speaking about the arrangements Marion had neglected to make for her children. Wald declared that a dying person who had evaded such a major responsibility could not be considered to have achieved true acceptance.

Because Klaus had begun to provide the bulk of the hands-on care Marion required, Wald had more time to interact with family members. Thus while Marion withdrew, Wald increased her commitment. Learning that Susanna had received all Ds on her report card and was unlikely to be admitted to any good college, Wald offered to use her connections to get Susanna into Wesleyan. When both Susanna and Helen told her that they needed part-time jobs, she tried to find employment for them at the hospital. One evening all three Weber girls as well as Susanna's new boyfriend had dinner at the Walds' house; later, Wald and her husband and daughter went with them to a high school concert. "The dinner was really very pleasant for us all," Wald reported, "a good deal of interchange."[46] As usual, she focused on psychological issues. Because Rose refused to relinquish the hope that her mother would recover, Wald attempted to orient her toward the truth. The girls' loving behavior continued to please. "The girls all greeted me very affectionately," Wald wrote after seeing them at the hospital. "Each one came up and kissed me."[47] After a phone call from Rose, she wrote, "There is a good deal of bantering and warmth and feeling back and forth between herself and myself."[48] Wald also felt closer to Susanna. Catching sight of her at the Black Panther Rally on May 1, Susanna ran to greet her. And Susanna too seemed to welcome Wald's ministrations. Finding her weeping in the hospital corridor after talking with her mother, Wald took Susanna to her office, where "she broke into deep sobs and I held her tightly in my arms while she cried unabashedly."[49]

In addition, Wald had the satisfaction of alleviating some of the tensions between Mrs. Klein and her granddaughters. Although Marion begged her mother not to upset the girls by continuing to prepare their meals, Rose complained that Klein came every day; recently they had had a fight, screaming loudly at each other. Marion recommended that Wald intervene, noting that "she was so tactful." A few days later, Wald went to the house around noon. Finding Klein making dinner, Wald tried to clean the dishes and otherwise "expedite things," so they could be gone by the time Rose returned from school. But Klein had the time wrong, and Rose arrived sooner than expected. After Wald explained why they were there, Rose "tried very hard not to start a fight." Wald then drove Klein to a Howard Johnson's, where they both got coffee and the grandmother had "a chance to express her feelings with less constraint."[50] She then confided her deep sadness about Marion and her many concerns about the girls and their futures.

The one relationship Wald could not resolve was hers with Alice. Wald readily agreed to perform another task that Alice considered distasteful: bringing the girls to view their mother's body if they wished to do so after she died. But new tensions arose. Alice had opposed the idea of sending her sister to the Hawkinses' home and remained resentful that Wald had prevailed. Wald suspected that because Alice had an "internal need" to act as a mother to her nieces, she was determined to bring them to her house despite their antipathy and would find a way to impose her will.[51] Although Wald prided herself on hiding her feelings from Alice, she freely expressed them in her case notes. She reported that after an especially unpleasant phone conversation, she had told her husband that Marion was a "bitch," conniving, and totally out of control.[52]

On the morning of May 30, Marion suddenly collapsed and was rushed to the hospital, where she died the following evening. Her last hours were miserable. Although she occasionally dozed, she "just grimaced and got mad and disgusted at her condition." Klaus could "almost hear her swearing under her breath." Now it was Goldenberg's turn to question Kübler-Ross's paradigm. Watching Marion "thrashing about" in the oxygen tent, he declared that the psychiatrist was "crazy." She had argued that adequate preparation would lead to a peaceful death. Whether or not Marion accepted her fate, she had received excellent care over several months and had been given many opportunities to express her emotions. Nevertheless, she endured terrible suffering at the end.[53]

The death initially seemed to heal the breach between Wald and Alice. Because Alice was at the hospital when Marion died and could not leave immediately, she asked Wald to go to the Weber house and tell the girls. When Alice arrived, Wald "felt at one with her—in helping the children express themselves and if something seemed funny, we were able to join them in laughing and if they were overwhelmed with grief, respond to this too." Later, Wald wrote, "Alice asked me if I could come to her house and be a member of the family with respect to the services and funeral on the following day, and I agreed to this."[54] But by the next day, their relationship had reverted to its usual form. Alice's behavior toward the Weber girls reinforced Wald's belief that their aunt should not take charge of them. Sitting next to Wald at the funeral, Rose put her head on Wald's shoulder and began to weep; Alice demanded that she sit up straight and stop crying. At the reception that followed at Alice's house, she insisted that Susanna and her friends, all about to graduate from high school, join the children in the basement. Later, Alice stated that she thought all three girls "needed to be brought in line." When her own children misbehaved, she not only reprimanded them but also slapped them, and she thought she should treat her nieces the same way.[55] Although Wald had coddled Rose, she especially needed the firm hand of Alice's husband.

Wald soon was prevented from intervening in any aspect of the girls' lives. Although she had vowed to stay in touch with them after their mother's death, she gradually realized that continuing involvement was counterproductive. As long as she participated in discussions about their future, Alice would resist compromise and demand that her nieces live with her. The issue remained unresolved when the girls left for a vacation with relatives in South Carolina, but Wald already had decided to withdraw. She explained that "while it was clear that the patient accepted me as a helper and a resource person and that the children also call me as helper and resource person, the sister has not seen me as such. In fact, an undercurrent of competition seems to have both Alice and myself in its clutches."[56] Replying to letters from the girls, she wrote that she wanted to remain helpful to them when and where she could but that arrangements on their behalf could be made more smoothly and easily in her absence. And indeed, when the girls returned to New Haven, they found that their relatives had followed the researchers' advice, hiring a young couple to live in their house.

Goldenberg now argued that the case could serve as a model. "There were a lot of intelligent, skilled people in the family, yet they were floundering about, really just spinning wheels, until [the research team] started engineering and organizing things. What happened is that our will was done, rather than what they wanted to do, [but] as it turned out, everybody is happy and relieved to have had a lot of decisions made." The Hirsches in particular were willing to follow the team's advice of hiring a couple because it "got them off the hook." The researchers were not just observing the study participants but also "contriving, engineering," and they noted that families seemed "to like this sort of thing."[57] That statement exposed the contradiction at the heart of Wald's enterprise. As in the previous case, she and her colleagues wanted both to understand the wants and needs of dying people and their families and to direct their behavior.

In September Wald wrote that she that she had regular contact with the girls. Later that month, she described a lunch with Rose. But Wald's attention soon shifted to other patients and families. She kept track of Marion's daughters primarily through Mrs. Klein, who reported that they were all doing well. Susanna had left for the University of Vermont, and both Helen and Rose liked the graduate history student and his wife who were caring for them. Although all three girls stopped by the Walds' house on New Year's Day 1970, Wald was no longer trying to sustain the relationship. When Rose asked if she could spend another weekend at the Walds' house in February, Wald discouraged her, and the girls' names soon disappeared from her notes.

Conclusion

Filling an enormous void in Marion Weber's life, Wald was able to forge a far more intimate relationship with her than she had with Nunzio Rossi. Many seriously ill people feel they have been banished from society, but Marion's sense of isolation must have been especially intense.[58] Before Wald's arrival, her only sources of support were a mother she detested and a sister preoccupied with her own life. In addition to offering concrete services, Wald showed that she was moved by Marion's suffering and assured her that her life still had meaning. The similarities between the two women strengthened their bond. Both were middle class, mothers of adolescent children, and Jewish.

Wald frequently argued that because death affected kin as well as patients, health professionals should care for all family members. Although she appears to have supported Marion's mother and daughters at especially critical times, she alienated Marion's sister. Ironically, the harshness of Wald's comments about Alice Hirsch can at least partly be explained by the fact that they too shared a cultural heritage, though with important variations. Opposed in principle to class privilege, Wald described Alice as the wrong kind of Jew—striving, wealthy, and shallow. Although we have less insight into Alice's point of view, we can assume she quickly perceived Wald's dislike and distrust. She also must have agreed that she and Wald inhabited different worlds and viewed Wald as an interloper, with too much power in her sister's life. By the end, she instinctively rejected any suggestion that came from Wald.

5

Making Sense of the Findings

Wald originally intended to publish a report of her study, laying the basis for the hospice she hoped to establish and educating the public about the experiences of patients and families confronting death. She relied heavily on Glaser and Strauss, who had pioneered what they termed *grounded theory* in their famous study of death and dying in hospitals. That methodology sought to derive theory by analyzing patterns, concepts, and themes that emerged from close observation of qualitative data. Wald found two presses that expressed interest in her work; consulted Jeanne Quint, a nurse who had worked closely with Glaser and Strauss; and met regularly with Diers, who taught classes on research methods. Despite Diers's constant encouragement, however, Wald rejected each of her own repeated attempts to generate categories from the diaries and transcripts. She labeled one version "trash" as soon as she finished it.[1]

One problem may have been confusion about the purpose of the study. Although Wald articulated her goal as understanding the wants and needs of dying people and their kin, she concentrated on needs, which she defined in therapeutic terms. She sought not only to gain insight into the experiences of the people she studied but also to encourage them to express their feelings about the approaching death. It was thus not entirely clear whether she should focus on what she learned about patients and families or on the extent to which she had been able to elicit the proper emotional response from them.

Wald later explained her inability to produce a publishable report by arguing that common social science concepts distorted the material. When she used the language of patients and caregivers, "the data fell easily into place," but she feared criticism from medical investigators. Having worked as a research assistant in medical facilities for several years, she was well aware of the criteria physicians used to assess different studies. She must have been especially discouraged by Goldenberg's comments that her sample was too small to produce valid information and that her data could receive "subjective analysis but not objective analysis."[2] In the end, she admitted defeat and turned her attention to planning the hospice. Now nearly half a century after Wald's attempt to analyze her research, it is possible to determine what her findings meant with less emotional involvement. In what follows, I draw inferences from the content of what she and her colleagues discovered and analyze the assumptions and values they brought to their work.

Attitudes toward Patients

Despite Wald's harsh criticism of Goldenberg's prejudices, she clearly had her own. Like a long line of health professionals before her, she repeatedly described Italian Americans as overly "emotional"; on at least one occasion, she used a common slur to refer to the Rossi family. Although her colleagues shared many of her views, they were more reluctant to act on the basis of imperfect knowledge. It is instructive to compare her attitude toward Italian and African Americans. As a supporter of the civil rights movement, she was extremely sensitive to any slights toward that group. She criticized Nunzio Rossi for firing a competent night nurse because she was black. Later she chastised herself when she met the well-dressed son of a patient and assumed he was a chauffeur. Perhaps because Italian Americans in the New Haven area opposed many local civil rights initiatives, Wald assumed they did not deserve the same courtesy.

But Italian Americans were not the only objects of her opprobrium. Her commitment to social justice also may explain why she always associated wealth with vanity, shallowness, and artificiality. A "superficial" woman, Ruth Cohen lacked the capacity to probe the painful emotions and existential issues raised by her proximity to death. Alice Hirsch's equally "superficial country-club household" disqualified her from serving as a guardian for her nieces. Within a decade, social scientists would begin to discuss the importance of "positionality"—the recognition that knowledge is always produced in a specific location and that biases may be introduced as a result.[3] In the late 1960s and early 1970s, however, few researchers interrogated their backgrounds or noted how preexisting assumptions might have colored their observations. Nevertheless, because Wald studied psychoanalysis, she might have been expected to apply contemporary theories about transference and countertransference. Those she appears to have ignored on several occasions.

Wald was more sensitive to the way personal preferences informed her actions. She took an immediate dislike to Sylvia Grand, a divorced woman who lived with her brother and his wife. Wald usually tried "to understand where the patient is at and adapt her interventions [accordingly]." But that technique was not appropriate for Grand, who "wanted to haul everyone down with her."[4] While other patients strove to sustain their independence, she seemed to revel in her dependence. Although Goldenberg agreed Grand was manipulative, he pointed out that she had advanced metastasis and must have felt extremely ill. Wald, however, remained convinced that Grand exaggerated her symptoms and could do much more for herself than she chose to admit. Much later, Wald acknowledged that Grand reminded her of her least favorite aunt.

From Cure to Care

Wald's emphasis on providing only palliative care to patients at the end of life was predicated on the assumption that it was possible to determine when curative treatment no longer would be effective and when patients wanted to stop fighting. After Nunzio was readmitted to the hospital, Wald argued that death was imminent and criticized the doctors for continuing to try one treatment after another. It is not clear, however, that she was more qualified than the doctors to estimate his prospect of survival or the utility of further therapy. He lived for six months after she pronounced him close to death. The rarity of his condition meant that no one knew his prognosis or an appropriate treatment. And given the language barrier, it was difficult to discern his wishes. Although he had chosen to leave the hospital despite knowing that home care might shorten his life, he may have felt differently after he returned.

A major reason the researchers decided to concentrate on patients with cancer diagnoses was that the disease's relatively predictable pattern made it easier to determine when death was likely to occur. But Wald was not sure she had made the correct call in the case of a woman with very advanced breast cancer. In chapter 2, I discussed Sofia Marsh, a fifty-eight-year-old teacher living with her daughter. She was gravely ill in April 1970 when she agreed to submit to an operation that promised to alleviate pain. It was a dangerous procedure for such a sick woman, and Marsh seemed near death during the two days that followed. Wald attributed Marsh's survival to the assiduous nursing care she herself had rendered. A few days later, she told her colleagues that she had had to make a "value judgment, an assessment, that this was a crisis situation but one in which [Marsh] hadn't given up the will to live." Now, however, Wald wondered if she had done "the right thing in trying to help her through." It had been "an almost superhuman task" to keep Marsh alive, and she had endured terrible suffering. "I put all this fight into it," Wald continued but admitted that she was "probably meeting my own needs as much as I was meeting hers."[5]

Because Wald viewed the Glaser and Strauss studies of hospital care for dying people as her "jumping off point," she decided not to focus on that topic in her own research. Nevertheless, she was incensed by what she observed. Preoccupation with curative treatments and medical research, she asserted, left no room for the solicitous care of people who were near death. Although Wald may have expected members of her own profession to display greater compassion than doctors, she complained about nurses who spoke in the past tense about patients who were still alive, made unpleasant remarks about dying people in their presence, or failed to respond to those in terrible pain.

Wald and her colleagues tried to educate hospital staff about the superiority of a new model of terminal care. They claimed some successes. Goldenberg reported that a few young doctors seemed receptive to his message. Wald and Klaus were pleased with an in-service training workshop they held for nurses on the ward. The most tangible victory concerned postmortem care. Although most hospitals provided little, if any, advice about how to care for dying people, nurses received extensive instructions about how to prepare a corpse.[6] Wald told her research team that she understood why most nurses feared death when she realized she was expected to take the clothes off the body of a woman she had known for several weeks, "put her on a plastic sheet, put that on top of the metal stretcher, rush her down to [the mortuary], unlock the ice-box, shove the stretcher in, bang the door shut, snap the lock and go upstairs and throw the chart on the admitting desk."[7] In a conference with a group of nurses, Wald complained about "that moment when the patient gives their last breath and suddenly becomes a piece of meat. That transition is very abrupt and isn't conducive to help us through the grieving process."[8] Soon afterwards, she reported that a hospital committee had accepted her recommendations for revising post mortem procedures.

Wald's disappointing interactions with medical staff during Nunzio's long stays, however, were typical of her efforts to transform hospital care for people before death occurred. Although she believed his doctors had an obligation to listen to her advice, they avoided her in the halls and excluded her from their rounds. Nunzio's nurses, she concluded, had no interest in the "humanistic" aspects of care. A medical student who observed Wald trying to "radicalize" the head nurse on a ward reported that the "nurse listened politely but was distant and cool."[9]

Because Wald wanted to study patients in nursing homes as well as hospitals, she and her colleagues sought information about those in the New Haven area. None provided the kind of care the researchers considered acceptable. The private residence Marion entered near the end of her life belonged to a vanishing group. Because most "mom and pop" nursing homes had difficulty complying with the regulations imposed by Medicare and Medicaid, larger, more medically oriented institutions had begun to replace them.[10] Although Goldenberg had encouraged Marion to go to Hawkins's home, he was appalled to find a total absence of nursing care, even for residents as gravely ill as Marion. Hawkins, in turn, complained that because Marion's family did not understand that she was in a home rather than an institution, they visited without asking permission and talked too loud. The fact that this was a residence rather than an institution also allowed her to be extremely selective in admissions. As noted in chapter 4, both a social worker and patient care coordinator noted that the facility was appropriate for someone "accustomed to gracious living." The researchers briefly considered applying to Hawkins on behalf of another woman before concluding she was not affluent enough to fit in. And soon the Hawkinses' home, like other "mom and pop" facilities, ceased to be an option for anyone. A few months after Marion's death, Hawkins's husband died, and she decided not to accept more residents.

The deficiencies of medical facilities heightened the attractiveness of home care. That also was the preference of patients and families. Marion insisted on staying home long after Goldenberg believed she should leave. Although Nunzio knew he could live longer in the hospital, both he and his wife demanded his discharge. But it was one thing to want a relative home during the days or weeks of a final illness and another to keep the patient home when death was imminent. "I think this is it," one man told Goldenberg, calling about his dying wife. The man then asserted that he "would rather she'd be in the hospital" because he felt "uncomfortable going through the night here."[11] The researchers asked two men whose wives had died in the hospital whether they would have preferred that death had occurred at home. Both adamantly declared that they were glad they had not been responsible for tending to their wives during the final hours.

Moreover, home care often entailed serious difficulties at any time. Soon after Nunzio arrived, Allegra appeared so tense that Wald feared she was prone to psychotic episodes. The wife of one son fled. When Nunzio returned to the hospital, he declared that he hoped never to inflict such a strain on his family again. Despite Marion's determination to remain with her daughters, she gained a sense of peace only after she left them. Financial difficulties compounded the problems. Nunzio's insurance money quickly evaporated. Marion could not afford to hire a housekeeper during the hours when one was most needed.

And many patients had little help from kin. A widow, Marion lived alone with her daughters and had only sporadic assistance from her mother and sister. Some married patients had spouses who had their own serious health conditions. A man with a heart problem, for example, could not lift his very obese wife. Although Wald and the other researchers did not mention the issue of gender, their records indicate that it was a major factor in several cases. Women historically have represented the great majority of family caregivers, but after Wald began to select study participants solely from Goldenberg's breast cancer clinic, all the spouses were men. Many had full-time employment. The husbands of two women had nine-to-five jobs in factories. One was not allowed to make phone calls during the day; the other occasionally had night shifts. The widespread belief that women alone had a duty to care may have been even more significant. Two women who relied heavily on husbands felt uncomfortable doing so and tried to lighten their burdens whenever possible. Two other women patients recalled that their brothers had absented themselves when their parents were ill. The women thus were not surprised when the men made no offers of to help them either. One was Sofia Marsh, whose brother lived four miles away but never visited and phoned only once during her last five months of life. John Strange, a recently retired man, provided hands-on care but horrified Klaus by grumbling incessantly about his burdens, usually in his wife's presence. He told Klaus he had retired because he wanted to fish; had he known he would have to spend his time tending a sick woman, he might have kept his job. Klaus "really felt badly" for the wife, although "she was smiling and being agreeable as he was complaining of the hardship she had put him through."[12]

Philippe Ariès argued that in the late nineteenth century, families began to exile dying patients to institutions to protect themselves from the unseemly aspects of death.[13] Although the extant records contain no examples of Wald encouraging relatives to enroll patients in hospitals for that reason, she discouraged discharge when she suspected that families would be exposed to sights and sounds they considered repellant. Cohen, for example, had assumed she would be able to rely on her mother when she left the hospital, but her doctor reported that "her chest wall malignancy [was] open and weeping and smelling and doing very poorly." Wald and her colleagues thus doubted the mother could handle the dressings. Wald wanted another woman to remain in the hospital for a similar reason: she had "a terribly big wound" that was "horrendous to see." Moreover, the fourteen-year-old daughter often shared a bed with her mother. "If I recoil and really even the doctors recoil from that dressing," Wald continued, it was difficult to imagine the girl sleeping near her mother. Wald also wanted to ensure that the seven-year-old daughter had no opportunity to witness her mother's death, which doctors predicted would be bloody and painful.[14]

When patients died at home, Wald and her colleagues sought to protect families from repellant sights. Despite her many criticisms of Alice Hirsch, Wald never faulted her for wanting to avoid providing intimate care for a sister with a large ulcerated wound. Nor did Wald question Alice's request that she not have to bring the Weber girls to visit their mother's body after her death. Although Strange's complaints about the burdens of care infuriated Klaus, her attitude softened when she realized how difficult it must be to bathe a "body so disfigured."[15] Wald and Klaus took pains to hide feelings of disgust from patients but were aware that they had little control over nonverbal cues. Both nurses tried to convince women that their lesions were neither as odorous nor as unsightly as the women feared. The nurses' facial expressions, however, often contradicted their words, undoubtedly intensifying patients' shame and humiliation.

Within a few years, hospice leaders would extol the virtues of home care. "The home is the natural place to die," declared a 1975 fund-raising appeal by Hospice Inc. "Protected from institutional encroachments upon their dignity, and thereby able to maintain individuality, the dying can avoid the isolation and anonymity that is too often their lot. They remain part of their family; they can participate, although in a limited way."[16] But at least some of the new emphasis on home care stemmed from financial constraints rather than patient and family preferences. The 1975 appeal noted that the average cost of hospital care for patients with advanced cancer was $21,718; for nearly a nearly a third, the cost was between $25,000 and $50,000. By providing most of their services outside institutions, hospices greatly reduced that enormous expense.[17] The passage of a hospice benefit under Medicare in 1983 rested not only on the argument that hospices offered a superior form of care but also on the contention that they saved money by relying on the "free" labor of families.[18] Today there is renewed pressure to shift more deaths out of institutions, compelling administrators and policy makers to disregard the issues Wald and her colleagues raised.

The study records demonstrate the difficulty of relying on physicians' comments to assess their level of honesty. Although Goldenberg assured a group of nurses that he always told the truth, he engaged in various forms of secrecy, especially about prognoses. But doctors were not the only ones to practice concealment. Marion refused to tell her daughters she was likely to die soon. Other women strove to remain in control of their lives, expending their last shreds of energy dressing themselves, eating meals at the table, and occasionally doing housework. Some also tried to manage their self-presentation when interacting with health care providers. Marion appears to have understood that her hysterical weeping in the hospital had violated what sociologists Glaser and Strauss referred to as the "sentimental order" of a hospital ward, "the intangible but very real patterning of mood and sentiment."[19] Even critically ill patients were expected to seem cheerful and optimistic. During the remainder of her stay, Marion strove to be the good patient. A week after her second outburst, one observer noted that she applied makeup and "put on a pleasant cheerful fun loving personality most of the time for the staff nurses."[20] After Wald remarked on Sofia Marsh's grayish complexion at home, Klaus reported that she "looks pretty good in the clinic" because there "she makes an effort to dress up and put on make-up."[21] Social proprieties further helped patients hide the severity of their conditions. One woman, for example, assumed that "fine" was the correct response when anyone asked how she was felt. Others took care not to cry in the presence of doctors.

Although both doctors and patients often had good reasons for using those various forms of concealment, deceit could have serious consequences. Some patients berated themselves for continuing to deteriorate after a doctor had assured them they could get better. Others lost trust in doctors who camouflaged the information that the patients knew experientially. Those who tried to hide advanced disease at home complained that family members refused to understand how sick they were and expected more from them than they possibly could give. Keeping up appearances was hard work, especially for gravely ill people.

Acceptance

Long after the Weber case closed, the researchers continued to debate the issues it had provoked about Kübler-Ross's theory. All members of the team agreed that she had identified the primary emotions dying people experienced, but some doubted that the different stages were distinct or followed an orderly sequence. Many patients seemed to move back and forth between stages or occupy several simultaneously. Other questions arose as well: Was it wrong to use medication or hypnosis to alleviate depression? Was that something patients had to work through? How could the researchers distinguish between denial and the confusion caused by a brain metastasis? Was a woman angry because she had to contemplate death or because her doctor had made a serious mistake?

Above all, the research team interrogated the meaning of acceptance. Revisiting the Weber case, Diers suggested that the researchers might never find an ideal version of acceptance, in the sense of a "beautiful rising up to heaven."[22] If they could break the notion into several component parts, they might be able to concentrate on the specific tasks Marion had been able to accomplish. Wald wondered if they had done something wrong by giving Marion ambiguous messages. Had they disguised the seriousness of her condition in an attempt to maintain hope? Both Wald and Klaus recalled several occasions on which they had tried to conceal how worried they were when dressing her lesion. The entire team tried to answer other thorny questions: Was it possible to encourage people to accept the inevitable without destroying hope? Did everyone have the potential to reach acceptance? Was it unrealistic to expect Marion to accept her mortality after sustaining so many other losses? Should they ever push patients into acceptance? Could they? And was the completion of unfinished emotional and practical business a prerequisite for gaining acceptance, as Wald insisted? Dobihal argued that no one had the right to define someone else's obligations. Wessel pointed out that everyone had some unfinished business.

Two later cases raised still other issues. In one, a declaration of acceptance by Kübler-Ross proved premature. On a visit to Yale in spring 1970, Kübler-Ross had interviewed Sofia Marsh and then concluded that she had passed through the first four phases of grief and arrived at the stage of acceptance. Klaus cautioned that Marsh's breast cancer still was at an early stage. Perhaps they should withhold judgment until they watched how she responded to the progression of her disease. And indeed, when Marsh began to complain in September, Klaus commented that she was "getting more *real*."[23] Visiting Marsh regularly during the last six months of her life, Klaus carefully observed her. Far from peacefully accepting the prospect of death, she was described as discouraged, angry, anxious, and depressed.

In the second case, the patient herself announced she had achieved equanimity. In December 1970, Susannah Post, a nurse, told Wald that after having had breast cancer for fifteen years, a third of her life, there was now "total acceptance of my part."[24] Wald had her doubts. Although Post had remained more active than other women with the same level of disease and spoke very openly about her condition, Wald had long wondered how much of her behavior was a performance. Now Wald pointed out that Post seemed very well defended against negative emotions. And it soon became clear that she had not reconciled herself to the end. When Post arrived at the clinic in February 1971, two months after making her pronouncement, Klaus missed her "big smile and sparkle." Post acknowledged that she had "reacted almost hysterically" to a recent bleeding episode, fearing it indicated a new metastasis. And she hoped Goldenberg would not prescribe more radiation because it was "devastating" to sit in the waiting room with so many dying people.[25]

Religion

The topic of religion was notable primarily by its absence in the records. Wald could not, of course, ignore the subject entirely. One of the first people she invited to join the research team was a Methodist minister. In addition, she recruited a young priest to talk to a woman she found especially difficult. When he left the parish, Wald found a substitute. She also noted that preparation for death had spiritual as well as emotional dimensions, that half of the study participants called themselves Catholic, and that clergy often visited them at home and in the hospital. In addition, she commented that the Rossis had a Madonna statue not only in Nunzio's hospital room but also on their front lawn, that religious pictures lined the walls of their house, and that Allegra sometimes spent the entire ride to the hospital saying her rosary.

But when a hospital nurse asked Wald how people drew on religious resources as they approached death, she had no response. She stressed that spirituality involved much more than belief in a divinity, that the counselling provided by the two priests was more psychological than religious, and that most clergy disappointed. One, for example, talked only about his eye problems when visiting a patient. Another stayed just a few minutes. Yet another priest delayed sending a letter to the Army to grant a soldier leave to see his mother before she died. At one point, Wald asked an anthropologist why a seemingly religious family like the Rossis seemed so antagonistic to priests, demanding that they leave Nunzio's room. When the anthropologist explained that deep religiosity among southern Italians often coexisted with fierce anticlericalism, Wald did not inquire about the meaning of that religiosity in the Rossi family life. In another case, Wald continually urged an Irish woman to talk openly about her feelings about death and dying. Explaining why the woman wished to be left alone, her fourteen-year-old daughter pointed out that, as Catholics, they had no problem accepting death because they viewed it as the way to go to heaven. Wald provided the name of a priest they could consult but continued to press the woman to express her emotions. Although Wald too placed a high value on acceptance, she believed it should come from psychological growth rather religious faith.

Wald understood that her attitude diverged sharply from that of Saunders. A committed Christian, Saunders viewed her hospice work as a personal calling and built St. Christopher's on a strong religious foundation. Although she welcomed patients with diverse affiliations, Anglican prayers were an essential part of the daily routine.[26] Visiting the facility in 1967, Wald found its "religious aspect hard to adjust to" because she was "not a religious person."[27] Many years later, Wald wondered if her group's lack of appreciation of religion had been "the basic flaw in our perception of hospice care from the beginning," and she expressed appreciation of Buddhism, with which her daughter, Shari, had become affiliated.[28] At the time of her study, however, Wald appeared almost totally indifferent to the role religion could play in helping terminally ill people come to terms with mortality. When Saunders visited the research team in 1970, Wald declared that in place of religion, the team was united by "working together in providing care to people who are in want. This seems to be enough."[29] Wald's views were shared by most, but not all, of the researchers. Returning from an eighteen-month sabbatical at St. Christopher's, Dobihal urged his American colleagues to follow Saunders's example and ensure that the hospice they planned had a firm religious orientation. Other members of the team vehemently disagreed.

Finances

Wald and Saunders not only disagreed about the place of religion in hospice care but also launched their facilities in very different contexts. As Goldenberg pointed out, British residents had received free medical care since the 1949 establishment of the National Health Service. The people he and Wald studied often faced serious financial issues that shaped medical decisions. Nunzio was fortunate to have Blue Cross, but he had to leave the hospital when he no longer could afford the deductible; he returned when he exhausted his coverage for home care. Marion was transferred to a tiny nursing home in part because she had difficulty paying the hospital fee.

Meeting for the first time just three years after Medicaid went into effect, the researchers were startled to discover that because the program was biased toward institutional care, it provided little funding for patients who wanted to remain at home. The program had other disadvantages as well. Because it was part of the welfare system, it stigmatized recipients and forced them to exhaust their funds in order to qualify. Wald and Klaus observed how Marsh confronted those issues during her last few months. By April 1971, it had become increasingly clear that she no longer could remain safely or comfortably at home without additional help. Although she lived with her daughter, she was busy with school and her fiancé and resented the burdens placed on her. Marsh could not afford to pay privately for home health care, and the local American Cancer Society rejected Klaus's request for financial help. But when Klaus suggested Marsh apply for Medicaid to enter a nursing home, she balked. As a nurse, she was familiar with horror stories about those facilities. She also did not want to receive Medicaid for reasons of pride and because she would have to relinquish her remaining income. In June Klaus reported that Marsh planned to pay out of pocket for home care until her funds ran out. In addition, "she planned on advertising in the free section of her town paper various things for sale: a tape recorder, hairdryer, dresses. She was a little shy to admit to these sales but obviously had thought a lot about it."[30]

With her health deteriorating and her daughter increasingly unwilling to help at the end of July, Marsh finally applied for Medicaid and entered a nursing home. Visiting her early in August, Wald reported that the staff could not meet the needs of the patients who "seemed almost like discarded bundles of clothes. . . . Three beds crowded into the one room-plus bedside furniture made it at best difficult to get around."[31] Klaus added that the "noisy patients around her upset her as well as their numerous families."[32] Medicaid, however, would not pay for a private room. Marsh died at the facility later that month.

If Wald felt inadequate preparing a professionally acceptable report of her findings, she displayed supreme confidence presenting them informally. No longer bound by the criteria of peer-reviewed publications, she took liberties with her material, carefully selecting the stories she wanted to tell and making generalizations on the basis of little or no evidence. We recall that, for example, the conflict in the Rossi family upset Wald, and some children failed to participate in the father's care. Handwritten notes she appears to have prepared for a talk gave this sentimentalized account: "In the home there was family solidarity that revolved around the father." Although the oldest son remained apart, "all the other children helped with family chores, plowing snow, canning tomatoes, building and repairing and of course preparing holiday meals."[33]

I have noted that Wald sought to facilitate the emotional growth of patients and families by encouraging them to express their feelings about mortality. Meeting with groups of nurses to educate them about her ideas, Wald ignored the many instances in which people had refused to disclose painful emotions; in other cases, she claimed success by fictionalizing events. One patient, for example, had "come through her dying process with a new stage of development."[34] But shortly before the woman died, Goldenberg had complained to the other researchers that "if ever I felt we have failed completely," it was with that patient. "At one point it appeared that she was willing to verbalize, to talk about her problems insofar as facing death is concerned." But then "she just closed up again, and continues to say, 'I'm going to be better tomorrow,' and 'I'm going to home tomorrow.' All the effort we put in to try to help her see what is going on has been completely for naught."[35] Wald too had grown discouraged. Visiting the woman at weekly intervals over several months, Wald had urged her to discuss her situation. But the patient remained silent, and Wald had begun to question whether such work ever could produce the desired results.

Klaus provided a detailed description of the agony another woman endured throughout her last day. Her body was so swollen that she could move only her head and hands. While Klaus and the patient's sister sat holding her hand, she began to mumble. When they asked what she was saying, she said she had not meant them to listen but was "just rambling on." At one point, she became more lucid and asked, "Why didn't you pull the plug while I was asleep last night?" She "kept repeating, pleading, looking me straight in the eye and saying, 'You could have, but you didn't.' She said, 'Oh, I wish I had the courage to kill myself.' The pain was in control, but every once in a while she would get very anxious and would need encouragement that she could breathe." Pain medication eventually helped her quiet down, but "her eyes bulged and she cried out a couple of times, 'Help me, help me, why can't you help me—do something.'" Finally, she slipped into a coma and died after half an hour.[36] Four days later, Wald told a group of nurses that she had worked with that woman for two weeks before she died. As a result, she was "able to verbalize very well exactly what she was going through and the fact that she was facing death and what the whole experience of dying meant to her." She described how "blackness began to enfold [her] and [about] losing sensation in her body, but her mind was completely alert until ½ hour before she took her last breath."[37]

Wald again embroidered the truth in a 1975 article she coauthored with another hospice nurse. A woman thinly disguised as Marion "was able to talk calmly and realistically of what would happen to her three teen-aged daughters" in the event of her death. During her weeks at a nursing home, "she was able to enjoy sunning herself in the garden, reading, and eating with gusto. All but the last five hours of her life were spent in rest and relaxation."[38] Although Marion may have talked to the girls in conversations that did not find their way into the notes, the extant records indicate that she failed to indicate that she failed to discuss the possibility of her death with the girls and plan for their future. Marion's suffering during her last day and a half was so terrible that Goldenberg began to wonder if anyone could have a peaceful death.

In addition, Wald made generalizations that that bore a striking resemblance to her initial assumptions but had little basis in fact. The 1975 article continued, "A nurses' hand, though full of skill is not the same as the hand of a loved one to mop a brow, rub a back, or touch an arm." We saw that Wald reported approvingly when Allegra brought special food to her husband and helped him bathe and go to the bathroom. But on the rare occasions Wald described a relative's care as having special meaning, she appears to have imputed feelings to the patient. Shortly before a woman died, she had asked her daughter to get her a particular kind of fudgsicle. Wald had been tempted to argue that the mother's swallowing was so bad she probably should not have the ice cream but then decided not to prevent the daughter "from meeting one of her mother's requests, something her mother wanted her to give, that she alone knew where to get, and that the hospital couldn't supply."[39] In another instance, Wald prided herself on showing a relative how to bestow care. A woman who visited her husband shortly before he died had found his "ability to respond was very slight." With Wald's encouragement, the wife held his hand. "At first, it had been difficult for her even to approach the bed and she sat perched on the edge of the chair. However, with a certain amount of encouragement and seeing that I could hold his hand, and that he seemed to enjoy this, she seemed to screw up her courage and did the same and it was very effective." Wald did not define what she meant by "effective."[40]

The 1975 article added that "a family's active participation in care . . . is part of the separation process itself, which includes giving and receiving, coming together, and letting go." Based on "clinical observations," Wald and her coauthor concluded that "family members who are involved in care are less prone to guilt and self-criticism." But on at least one occasion, Wald may have seen things that were not there. After praising the "remarkable" amount of care two sisters gave a dying patient, Wald commented that their work would "help the bereavement process very much." Visiting the two women at the funeral home, she observed "a kind of quiet sadness, but you really had a feeling that a lot of the emotional crises have been worked through."[41] She knew nothing, of course, about how the women actually felt or how they fared in the weeks and months ahead.

Wald also told a group of nurses that she had "noticed that patients who had unfinished business, especially with regard to children or other dependents, had a more difficult time letting go of life" than others.[42] It is true that Wald had often encouraged Marion to make plans for her daughters and promised she might die more easily if she did so. But there is no evidence that Marion's failure to fulfill that responsibility led her to cling to life more tenaciously or caused more suffering when she died.

Wald was able to point to one case that seemed to substantiate her claim. A woman who had participated in the study died peacefully in her sleep just after completing all the necessary practical arrangements. In this instance, Wald asserted a causality she could not prove. In addition, she ignored the immense amount of time and attention the patient had consumed. Wald first met Carmela Moretti, a sixty-four-year-old Italian American woman with terminal breast cancer, in January 1970. Finding her anxious and depressed, Wald referred her to a psychiatrist and spoke to her "almost daily" until March, when she decided a priest might be more helpful.[43] Father Don McNeil then met with Moretti weekly for several months. Because their hour-long conversations were tape recorded and transcribed, we have access to their content. McNeil must have found the sessions extremely frustrating. Moretti talked on and on, paying little attention to his comments and repeating the same grievances over and over. Her primary complaint focused on her husband from whom she was separated. Although he lived three blocks away, he never called or visited. She believed she had wasted the forty years she had spent with him because she was now so lonely. Her three grown children visited on weekends, but she spent many days with little or no company. When McNeil left the parish, Father Canny, a member of the research team, replaced him, and the meetings continued. Shortly before Moretti's death in August, she divided her property among her children and seemed somewhat more reconciled to her fate.

Nevertheless, the case could not serve as a model. Few institutions of any kind could devote so much attention to a single individual.

It is tempting to argue that yet another reason Wald had such difficulty preparing an academic report is that she had a particular story she wanted to tell. "Your *alter* country is everything that your first is not," writes the English author Julian Barnes. "Commitment to it involves idealism, love, sentimentality, and a certain selective vision."[44] Wald's other country was the hospice she planned to establish. She undoubtedly assumed she could enlist the support of others only if she could demonstrate that the terminal care delivered in a hospice would be better in every way than that provided in a hospital. That goal required selectivity and embellishment.

Conclusion

When Hospice Inc. (soon renamed the Connecticut Hospice) opened in New Haven in 1975, Florence Wald was appointed director. Soon, however, the board of directors began to receive complaints from staff members that she tried to insert herself into every aspect of their work, and after a year, she was asked to resign. Nevertheless, she remained actively involved in the hospice movement, traveling frequently to promote the establishment of programs throughout the country. In the 1990s, she joined the board of the National Prison Hospice Association, which trained inmates to serve as hospice volunteers within state correctional facilities. She explained that the hospice model was especially important for prison inmates because they often felt a sense of failure about their lives. In addition, the volunteers gained confidence, showing "that even in this terrible situation, something good can happen, a sense of possibility emerges."[1] Although Wald's tenure at Hospice Inc. was brief, her extraordinary contribution to its creation won recognition. She was awarded an honorary degree from Yale University, inducted into the National Women's Hall of Fame, and named a Living Legend by the American Academy of Nursing. She died at the age of ninety-one in 2008.

Edward F. Dobihal played a major role in establishing Hospice Inc. and served as the first chair of its board of directors. Later he was instrumental in founding both a New Haven halfway house for people with mental illness and a group dedicated to helping elderly Hamden residents stay in their homes. His coauthored book *When a Friend Is Dying: A Guide to Caring for the Terminally*

Ill and Bereaved appeared in 1984.[2] He remained director of the department of religious ministries at Yale New Haven Hospital (YNHH) and associate clinical professor at Yale Divinity School until 1990, when he became pastoral consultant to the Yale School of Nursing and the department of religious ministries at YNHH. He also continued to participate actively in the civil rights and peace movements.[3] He retired from Yale in 1989 and died in 2015.

Despite Wald's fears that Ira S. Goldenberg would lose interest in her project, he was a leading member of the group planning Hospice Inc. and later served as the vice chair of the board of directors. In a 1979 article in the *Bulletin of the American College of Surgeons*, he wrote that the hospice "is a reaffirmation of all the precepts of good medical care that physicians have been practicing for generations. These precepts sometimes become lost in the maze of modern medical practice, but they must become prominent again."[4] Until his death from a heart attack at fifty-seven in 1982, he remained a clinical professor of surgery at Yale Medical School. He was an early advocate of replacing the radical mastectomy with less mutilating surgery.[5] A 2012 history of the cancer program at Yale referred to him as one of the clinical professors who had made major contributions to cancer treatment.[6]

Morris Wessel was another leader of the group responsible for establishing Hospice Inc. Throughout his career, he continued to be deeply concerned about bereaved children and adolescents. His article, "A Death in the Family: The Impact on Children," appeared in the *Journal of the American Medical Association* in 1975. In addition, he was one of the first pediatricians to point out the dangers of lead poisoning in children. When he retired in 1993, hundreds of family members, former patients, and friends attended a celebration of his life in a New Haven park. A *New York Times* article about the event described him as "a much-loved New Haven doctor."[7] The same year, he received the American Academy of Pediatrics Practitioner Research Award. He died in 2016.

When Wald's study ended, Katherine Klaus worked briefly on the committee planning the new hospice before concluding that she did not want to become involved in the politics surrounding it. She devoted the rest of her career to school nursing.[8]

Donna Diers remained on the faculty of the Yale University School of Nursing, serving as dean from 1972 to 1985. The author of numerous academic articles on nursing and health policy, she was editor of *Image: Journal of Nursing Scholarship* for eight years. In the 1970s, she was a member of the Yale group that classified hospital cases into diagnosis-related groups; that research laid the basis for the prospective payment system instituted by Medicare. In 1910, the American Academy of Nursing named her a Living Legend. After her death in 2013, numerous nursing leaders and former students wrote testimonials describing her as a pioneering researcher and devoted mentor and teacher.[9]

The study in which these individuals participated expands our understanding of U.S. hospices. Like Wald's articles and talks about her research findings, most early accounts of hospice services glorified them by telling carefully selected stories.[10] The great advantage of Wald's extensive notes is that they enable us to glimpse the complexities those stories conceal. "One of the basic tenets of hospice care is the treatment of patient and family together," wrote Robert W. Buckingham, a professor of family and community medicine who had been research director of Hospice Inc. in 1983. Hospice leaders censured hospital regulations that disrupted intimate ties just when the need for them was greatest. Because most ICUs limited visits to five minutes an hour, patients often died alone with the family banished to the waiting room. By contrast, Buckingham stated, "Hospice helps to make death a coming together." The staff is trained "to facilitate communication between family members so that the remaining time can be as complete as possible. Family problems cannot be ignored, for if they remain unresolved they affect the peace of the dying person. When family members are able to express feelings, patients feel less isolated and freer to express their feelings."[11]

Promoting family harmony proved more difficult than Wald had anticipated. She liked some patients and relatives and disliked others. It is likely that, given her own antipathy to Alice Hirsch and her husband, Wald did not even attempt to convince the Weber girls to consider them their guardians. Nor could she overcome the cleavages within the Rossi family. She stated that she reconciled one son with his wife, but she does not appear to have strengthened the bond between Nunzio and Allegra. When Wald tried to heal the breach between Nunzio and Robert, one of her long-standing goals, both turned their ire on her.

One problem was that sickness often ignited family tensions. As a result of the various conflicts Nunzio's care had precipitated, Robert was more alienated from the rest of the family than he had been at the beginning of the case. When Marion Weber became too ill to run her household on her own, her mother came to cook and clean. Mrs. Klein's presence, however, exacerbated ongoing tensions between herself and her daughter and granddaughters. Another problem was that Wald interpreted facilitating communication as encouraging patients and family members to express their feelings and share them with each other. Such a notion was alien to many study participants.

Home care was another element of the hospice vision. "Most patients wish to stay at home as long as they can, to die at home if possible," wrote clergyman Parker Rossman in 1977. "Keeping the dying person home also . . . enables the terminally ill to escape institutional encroachments upon their dignity, to avoid the isolation and autonomy which is so often their lot, and makes it possible for them to continue sharing in the life of their family."[12] Buckingham added that children as well as adults should be able to "witness the dying process at home, and not be frightened by it. A positive experience at home can counteract the unnatural scenes of violent death that saturate the media."[13]

On that issue, Wald appears to have held reservations. Although she agreed that hospitals were not good places for most dying people, she shared the fears of Nunzio's doctor and nurse about sending him back to a family that seemed unlikely to deliver good care. She also catalogued the problems generated by Nunzio's arrival home. Allegra collapsed emotionally from the strain of caring for him. When the insurance coverage expired, none of the family members felt qualified to change his IV. Without adequate nursing care, he developed a fever. Marion's experience also provided a cautionary tale. Although she was determined to remain at home even as her health steadily deteriorated, she began to find her daughters' demands and commotion intolerable. She gained a sense of peace only when she was able to live apart from them.

In yet another case, Wald wanted a woman to remain in the hospital to relieve her fourteen-year-old daughter of responsibility for her care. Moreover, far from believing that everyone could have a positive experience witnessing death, Wald was aware that some deaths were far from peaceful and that children needed to be protected from the sight of them. "A change in setting, hospital to home, brought a sense of freedom," Wald later wrote. "When symptoms were out of control, family relations became tangled, or when we felt unsure of ourselves, however, the hospital felt safer than home."[14] Some family members in the study asked that hospitals readmit patients who were on the verge of death.

Early hospices also placed a high premium on honesty. As Wald frequently emphasized, patients could prepare for mortality only if they knew it was near. Accurate and complete information also was essential to patient autonomy. Even people closest to death, hospice leaders asserted, could retain a sense of personal mastery by exercising authority over their care. It was common to assess the level of physician honesty by asking doctors about their practices, but that method might not have produced reliable information. Despite his avowed commitment to telling the truth, Goldenberg followed most of his colleagues in concealing poor prognoses. Two nurses who worked with Wald condemned secrecy in general but justified some of Goldenberg's practices, noting that many patients did not want to learn the full details of their conditions. And although Wald's commitment to honesty never faltered, she occasionally found herself shading the truth.

Teamwork also had a central place in the hospice mission. Because the first step in care of dying patients was to control pain and other symptoms, medical expertise was essential. But hospice proponents pointed out that human life was more than "a breathing lung and beating heart": people at the end of life had emotional, social, and spiritual needs, not just physical problems.[15] Although doctors directed the activities of other staff in hospitals, a physician employed by a hospice program was regarded as one among a number of equal members of an interdisciplinary team and had no automatic entitlement to the position of leader. Wald's relationship with Goldenberg demonstrated how difficult it was to achieve that goal. When Wald designated Goldenberg as the primary doctor on her research team, she was convinced she had found one of the few hospital doctors who would agree to work with nurses as equals. Goldenberg quickly disabused her of that notion, insisting that he alone would make decisions regarding his patients' care. Although warm and solicitous of his patients, he often appeared arrogant and overbearing in interactions with Wald. When she urged a woman to repeat a question Goldenberg had failed to answer, he reprimanded her harshly.

Finally, hospices emphasized the importance of accepting mortality as a part of life. Viewing death as a natural event rather than a technological failure, they condemned the curative focus of modern medicine. Above all, they asserted that dying individuals must find a way to accept their fragility.[16] I have argued that the hope and optimism prescribed by contemporaneous cancer organizations increased the denial surrounding death and denigrated dying people. Wald offered those under her care a very different framework for understanding their plights. Rather than suggesting that people had the power to stave off death by maintaining strict surveillance over their bodies, she pointed to life's inherent fragility. And rather than avoiding the topic of mortality, she encouraged individuals to summon the resources needed to confront its stark reality. When Kübler-Ross's *On Death and Dying* appeared in November 1969, the month Marion entered the Yale study, Wald and her colleagues tried to apply the book's theory to their findings. Psychological growth now meant passing through various emotional stages to reach acceptance, the prerequisite for a peaceful death. Nevertheless, acceptance proved as elusive as recovery. Despite their many attempts, the researchers failed to find an example of a woman whose experience matched Kübler-Ross's paradigm. Nor could they always determine when death was inevitable and aggressive treatment no longer effective.

But if the records of Wald's study indicate that hospices could not possibly fulfill the inflated ideals they proclaimed, the records also demonstrate that since the beginning of the hospice movement, it has provided a radical alternative to protracted and brutal hospital deaths. Wald and her colleagues sought to respond sensitively to the suffering of dying patients, enable them to remain close to the most important people in their lives, and protect them from futile and aggressive therapies. The many programs based on Wald's principles similarly countered the technological, curative focus of modern medicine, inspiring others to try to transform care for people at the end of life. And still today, patients and family members throughout the country laud hospice staff members who deliver care with extraordinary warmth and compassion.

The greatest threat to the hospice ideal is no longer pressure for accommodation to the established health care system but rather a growing concern with the bottom line. Most observers agree that Congress made hospices a Medicare benefit in 1982 in order to contain health care costs. The early years of the Reagan administration were a time of economic retrenchment. Growing popular support for hospice ideals undoubtedly facilitated passage of the benefit, but that outcome was ensured by a Congressional Budget Office report concluding that the government could save as much as $1,120 for each Medicare beneficiary enrolled in hospice.[17] The savings were to come from reliance on unpaid kin. To ensure that care shifted from hospital to home, the legislation limited the number of inpatient days a hospice could provide to 20 percent of the total Medicare patient days. While Wald and her colleagues sought to treat family members as well as patients with solicitude and relieve the most onerous caregiver burdens, kin now increasingly are viewed simply as a form of cheap labor. And family caregiving has become increasingly difficult. In the years since Allegra and her children quailed at the idea of changing Nunzio's IV, many other technologies have been adapted for the home. Family members now are expected to perform a broad array of complex nursing and medical tasks that previously were the exclusive province of health professionals.

The rejection of patients who require chemotherapy and radiation also illustrates the growing dominance of a business ethos. That policy stems in part from history: throughout the 1970s and 1980s, those therapies were administered only when they offered some promise of cure. But the line between curative and palliative treatments has faded; physicians now use chemotherapy and radiation to improve the quality of life of terminally ill patients. The primary disadvantage of the treatments today, many commentators charge, is their expense. In addition, hospices increasingly discharge patients before death. In some cases, the patients may have improved or decided to resume curative treatment. In others, however, the motive is to avoid paying for costly medical care. Although those practices exist throughout the hospice industry, they are especially common in for-profit entities. More than half of all hospices are profit-making today, and many of those are attached to large chains.[18] Referring to the extremely high discharge rate of for-profit programs, one prominent researcher recently commented that "you have to wonder" if they are "living up to the vision and morality of their founders."[19]

In short, Wald's study both demonstrates that some of the original hospice ideals were unattainable and describes a model of compassionate care that can be easily betrayed.

Notes

Introduction

1. Florence and Henry Wald Papers (MS 1659) Manuscripts and Archives, Yale University Library, New Haven, Connecticut. Two dissertations that discuss the study are Joy Buck, "Rights of Passage: Reforming Care of the Dying, 1965–1986" (PhD diss., University of Virginia, 2005), and Cynthia C. Adams, "Dying with Dignity in America: The Transformational Leadership of Florence Wald" (EdD diss., University of Hartford, 2008).

2. Emily K. Abel, "The Hospice Movement: Institutionalizing Innovation," *International Journal of Health Services* 16, no. 1 (1986): 71–85.

3. Nicky James and David Field, "The Routinization of Hospice: Charisma and Bureaucratization," *Social Science and Medicine* 34, no. 12 (1992): 1363–95.

4. David Clark, "Hospice Care of the Dying," in *Death, Dying, and Bereavement: Contemporary Perspectives, Institutions, and Practices*, ed. Judith M. Stillion and Thomas Attig (New York: Springer, 2015), 135–49.

5. Joel Wald, telephone interview, January 20, 2017.

6. Donald Oken, "What to Tell Cancer Patients: A Study of Medical Attitudes," *JAMA* 175, no. 13 (April 1, 1961): 86–94.

7. Dennis H. Novack, Robin Plumer, Raymond L. Smith, Herb Omegert Ochitill, Gary R. Morrow, and John M. Bennett, "Changes in Physicians' Attitudes toward Telling the Cancer Patient," *JAMA* 241, no. 9 (March 2, 1979): 897–900. See Sydney A. Halpern, "Medical Authority and the Culture of Rights," *Journal of Health Politics, Policy and Law* 29, nos. 4–5 (August–October 2004): 835–52; Anne Harrington, *The Cure*

Within: A History of Mind-Body Medicine (New York: W. W. Norton, 2008); Mary Ann Krisman-Scott, "Historical Analysis of Disclosure of Terminal Status," *Image* 32, no. 1 (2000): 47–52; David J. Rothman, *Strangers at the Bedside* (New Brunswick: Transaction, 1991); Carl E. Schneider, *The Practice of Autonomy: Patients, Doctors, and Medical Decisions* (New York: Oxford University Press, 1998); Robert Zussman, "Sociological Perspectives on Medical Ethics and Decision-Making," *Annual Review of Sociology* 23 (1997): 171–89.

8. O. G. Brim, H. E. Freeman, S. Levine, and N. A. Scotch, *The Dying Patient* (New York: Russell Sage Foundation, 1970); Rosemary Stevens, *In Sickness and in Wealth: American Hospitals in the Twentieth Century* (New York: Basic Books, 1989), 231.

9. Julie Fairman and Joan Lynaugh, *Critical Care Nursing: A History* (Philadelphia: University of Pennsylvania Press, 1998), 2.

10. See *Final Report of the Advisory Committee on Human Radiation Experiments* (New York: Oxford University Press, 1996); Ezekiel J. Emanuel, Christine Grady, Robert A. Crouch, Reidar K. Lie, Franklin G. Miller, and David Wendler, eds., *The Oxford Textbooks of Clinical Research Ethics* (New York: Oxford University Press, 2008).

11. Drew Gilpin Faust, *This Republic of Suffering: Death and the American Civil War* (New York: Knopf, 2008), 31.

Chapter 1. Setting the Stage

Unless otherwise indicated, all files are from the Florence and Henry Wald Papers, MS 1659, Manuscripts and Archives, Sterling Memorial Library, New Haven, CT.

1. Monica Mills, "Interview with Florence Wald," Oral History Archive, Connecticut Women's Hall of Fame, June 10, 2003.

2. Florence Wald, "The Emergence of Hospice Care in the United States," in *Facing Death*, ed. Howard M. Spiro, Mary G. McCrea Curnen, and Lee Palmer Wandel (New Haven: Yale University Press, 1996), 81–89.

3. Mills, "Interview."

4. Mills.

5. Florence Wald, "In Search of the Spiritual Component of Hospice Care," in *In Quest of the Spiritual Component of Care for the Terminally Ill: Proceedings of a Colloquium, May 3–4, 1986*, Yale University School of Nursing, ed. Florence S. Wald (New Haven: 1986), 25. Copyright Florence S. Wald.

6. Cynthia Connolly, personal interview, Philadelphia, May 4, 2017.

7. Shari Wald Vogler, phone interview, February 14, 2017.

8. Elizabeth Fee, "The Origins of Public Health Nursing: The Henry Street Visiting Nurse Service," *American Journal of Public Health* 100, no. 7 (July 2010): 1207.

9. Quoted in Joy Buck, "Rights of Passage: Reforming Care of the Dying, 1965–1986," (PhD diss., University of Virginia, 2005), 89.

10. "Curriculum Vitae, Florence S. Wald," File 2. In 2003, the name of Babies Hospital was changed to the NewYork-Presbyterian Morgan Stanley Children's Hospital.

11. Quoted in Jed S. Rakoff, "Neuroscience and the Law: Don't Rush In," *New York Review of Books*, May 12, 2016.

12. Wald, "Emergence of Hospice Care," 82.

13. Barbara J. Callaway, *Hildegard Peplau: Psychiatric Nurse of the Century* (New York: Springer, 2002), 261.

14. Hildegard E. Peplau, *Interpersonal Relations in Nursing: A Conceptual Frame of Reference for Psychodynamic Nursing* (New York: Springer, 1991); See Patricia D'Antonio, Linda Beeber, Grayce Sills, and Madeline Naegle, "The Future in the Past: Hildegard Peplau and Interpersonal Relations in Nursing," *Nursing Inquiry* 21, no. 4 (2014): 311–17.

15. Cynthia Connolly, personal interview, January 30, 2017.

16. Mills, "Interview."

17. Donna Diers, "Before Hospice: Florence Wald at the Yale School of Nursing," *Illness, Crisis, and Loss* 17, no. 4 (2009): 309.

18. Diers, "Before Hospice," 309. See Helen Varney Burst, "Yale School of Nursing: Celebrating 90 Years of Excellence," *Yale School of Nursing Alumni Newsletter and Magazines*, 2013, http://elischolar.library.yale.edu/ysn_alumninews/182.

19. Virginia A. Henderson, *The Nature of Nursing: Reflections after 25 Years* (New York: Macmillan, 1966), 10.

20. Henderson, *Nature of Nursing*, 25.

21. Henderson.

22. David Clark, "'Total Pain,' Disciplinary Power and the Body in the Work of Cicely Saunders, 1958–1967," *Social Science and Medicine* 49 (1999): 727–36.

23. Mills, "Interview."

24. "Biographical Data—Edward F. Dobihal, Jr.," File 2.

25. Morris Wessel, "Social Action as Spiritual Component: The Relevance of Nicaragua," in *In Quest of the Spiritual Component of Care for the Terminally Ill: Proceedings of a Colloquium, May 3–4, 1986, Yale University School of Nursing*, ed. Florence S. Wald (New Haven: 1986), 141. Copyright Florence S. Wald.

26. "Curriculum Vitae, Morris A. Wessel," File 2.

27. James Sullivan, "Dr. Freud and Dr. Spock," *The Courier* (1995), http://surface.syr.edu/libassoc/328.

28. Nancy Polk, "A Much-Loved New Haven Doctor Retires," *New York Times*, July 23, 1993.

29. Morris Wessel, "He Gave Me Courage," *Yale Alumni Magazine*, Summer 1998.

30. Sara Lee Silberman, "Edith Banfield Jackson," in *Notable American Women*, ed. Susan Ware and Stacy Baukman, vol. 5 (Boston: Belknap Press, 2005), 323–24; Sara Lee Silberman, "Pioneering in Family-Centered Maternity and Infant Care: Edith B. Jackson and the Yale Rooming-In Research Project," *Bulletin of the History of Medicine* 64, no. 2 (Summer 1990): 262–87; Elizabeth Temkin, "Rooming-In: Redesigning Hospitals and Motherhood in Cold War America," *Bulletin of the History of Medicine* 76, no. 2 (Summer 2002): 271–98; Morris A. Wessel and Frederic M. Blodgett, "Edith B. Jackson, M. D. and Yale Pediatrics," *Connecticut Medicine* 26, no. 7 (July 1962): 438–41.

31. Wessel, "Social Action," 142.

32. "Ira S. Goldenberg, Curriculum Vitae," 1968, File 2.

33. Sherwin B. Nuland, *Lost in America: A Journey with My Father* (New York: Random House, 2003), 174–75.

34. Nuland, *Lost in America*, 198–99.

35. Katherine Klaus, personal interview, North Haven, Connecticut, November 28, 2016.

36. Sharon Eck Birmingham and Suzanne M. Boyle, "A Legacy of Data Use by Donna Diers," *Nursing Economics* 31, no. 3 (May/June 2013): 144; Diana J. Mason, "In Memoriam: Donna Diers," *American Journal of Nursing* 113, no. 4 (April 2013): 19; Colleen Shaddox, "A Former Dean, But Never a Former Nurse," *Yale Alumni Magazine*, May/June 2013.

37. Mills, "Interview."

38. Jennifer Nelson, *More than Medicine* (New York: New York University Press, 2015).

39. Randi Hutter Epstein, *Get Me Out: A History of Childbirth from the Garden of Eden to the Sperm Bank* (New York: W. W. Norton, 2010), 128.

40. John Case and Rosemary C. R. Taylor, eds., *Co-ops, Communes, and Collectives: Experiments in Social Change in the 1960s and 1970s* (New York: Pantheon Books, 1979).

41. "Conference," September 13, 1969, File 14.

42. Norman I. Fainstein and Susan S. Fainstein, "New Haven: The Limits of the Local State," in *Restructuring the City: The Political Economy of Urban Redevelopment*, ed. Susan S. Fainstein, Norman I. Fainstein, Richard Child Hill, Dennis R. Judd, and Michael Peter Smith (New York: Longman, 1983), 27–79; Mandi Isaacs Jackson, *Model City Blues: Urban Space and Organized Resistance in New Haven* (Philadelphia: Temple University Press, 2008).

43. "Knowledge Center: Supportive Community Governance through Collaborative Knowledge, Data and Analysis," DataHaven, accessed July 30, 2016, http://www.ctdatahaven.org/sites/ctdatahaven/files/know/index.

44. Mills, "Interview."

45. Warren Goldstein, *William Sloane Coffin, Jr., A Holy Impatience* (New Haven: Yale University Press, 2004), 183.

46. Amy Vita Kesselman, "Women's Liberation and the Left in New Haven, Connecticut, 1968–1972," *Radical History Review*, no. 81 (Fall 2001): 17.

47. Quoted in Joy Buck, "'I Am Willing to Take the Risk': Politics, Policy, and the Translation of the Hospice Ideal," *Journal of Clinical Nursing* 18, no. 19 (October 2009): 2704.

48. "The Rev. Edward Dobihal," *Impact, Yale–New Haven Hospital* (Summer 2009): 14.

49. Diers, "Before Hospice," 308.

50. Diers, 311.

51. Elisabeth Kübler-Ross, *On Death and Dying* (New York: Scribner, 1969).

52. Quoted in Holcomb B. Noble, "Elisabeth Kübler-Ross, 78, Dies; Psychiatrist Revolutionized Care of the Terminally Ill," *New York Times*, August 26, 2001.

53. Joy Buck, "Reweaving a Tapestry of Care: Religion, Nursing, and the Meaning of Hospice, 1945–1978," *Nursing History Review* 15 (2007): 133.

54. Stephanie Coontz, *A Strange Stirring: The Feminine Mystique and American Women at the Dawn of the 1960s* (New York: Basic Books, 2001), 145.

55. See Clifton D. Bryant, "The Sociology of Death and Dying," in *21st Century Sociology: A Reference Handbook*, ed. Clifton D. Bryant and Dennis L. Peck (Newbury Park: Sage, 2007), 157.

56. Henry Feifel, "Introduction," in *The Meaning of Death*, ed. Henry Feifel (New York: McGraw-Hill, 1959), xiv.

57. Jessica Mitford, *The American Way of Death* (New York: Simon and Schuster, 1963).

58. Bryant, "Sociology of Death and Dying."

59. Robert Fulton, ed., *Death and Identity* (New York: John Wiley and Sons, 1965), ix.

60. Barney G. Glaser and Anselm L. Strauss, *Awareness of Dying* (New Brunswick: Aldine Transaction, 1965); Barney G. Glaser and Anselm L. Strauss, *Time for Dying* (New Brunswick: Aldine Transactions, 1968); David Sudnow, *Passing On* (Englewood Cliffs: Prentice-Hall, 1967); Jeanne C. Quint, *The Nurse and the Dying Patient* (New York: Macmillan, 1967).

61. "Way of Dying," *Atlantic Monthly*, January 1957, 53.

62. "A New Way of Dying," *Reader's Digest*, March 1957.

63. Joseph Fletcher, "The Patient's Right to Die," *Harper's Magazine*, October 1960, 143.

64. Paul Ramsey, *The Patient as Person: Explorations in Medical Ethics*, 2nd ed. (New Haven: Yale University Press, 2002), 116–64.

65. "Life-in-Death," *New England Journal of Medicine* 256 (April 18, 1957): 760.

66. Frank J. Ayd Jr., "The Hopeless Case: Medical and Moral Considerations," *Journal of the American Medical Association* 181, no. 13 (September 19, 1962): 1100; for other works by physicians who questioned the

tendency to prolong life even after the possibility of recovery became slim in the early 1960s, see Thomas T. Jones, "Dignity in Death: The Application and Withholding of Interventive Measures," *Journal of the Louisiana State Medical Society* 113, no. 5 (May 1961): 180–83; James A. Knight, "Philosophic Implications of Terminal Illness," *North Carolina Medical Journal* 22, no. 10 (October 1961): 493–95.

67. Edward H. Rynearson, *CA: A Cancer Journal for Clinicians* 9, no. 3 (May/June 1959): 85.

68. Leland Christenson, "Editorial: The Physician's Role in Terminal Illness and Death," *Minnesota Medicine* 46 (September 1963): 881.

69. John B. Graham, "Acceptance of Death—Beginning of Life," *North Carolina Medical Journal* 24, no. 5 (August 1963): 317.

70. Knight, "Philosophic Implications," 495.

71. See Samuel Standard and Helmuth Nathan, eds., *Should the Patient Know the Truth* (New York: Springer Publishing, 1955).

72. Louis Lasagna, "Editorial: The Doctor and the Dying Patient," *Journal of Chronic Diseases* 22 (1969): 66.

73. See William Kitay, "Let's Retain the Dignity of Dying," *Today's Health* (May 1966): 62–69.

74. Charles Bosk, *Forgive and Remember: Managing Medical Failure*, 2nd ed. (Chicago: Chicago University Press, 2003).

75. Glaser and Strauss, *Time for Dying*.

76. Glaser and Strauss, *Awareness of Dying*.

77. Quint, *Nurse and the Dying Patient*, 11.

78. Barbara Melosh, *"The Physician's Hand": Work, Conflict, and Culture in American Nursing* (Philadelphia: Temple University Press, 1982), 56.

79. Jeanne C. Quint, "Awareness of Death and the Nurse's Composure," *American Journal of Nursing* 15, no. 1 (Winter 1966): 49–55.

80. Wilma R. Lewis, "A Time to Die," *Nursing Forum* 4 (1965): 9.

81. Mary Catherine Short Googe, "The Death of a Young Man," *American Journal of Nursing* 64, no. 11 (November 1964): 133.

82. Dorothy Whitehouse, "Johnny—The Little Boy Who Never Smiled," *American Journal of Nursing* 55, no. 9 (September 1955): 1110.

83. Mary L. Knipe, "Serenity for a Terminally Ill Patient," *American Journal of Nursing* 66, no. 10 (October 1966): 2254.

84. Patricia Reimer, Lee Rouse Bone, and Rebecca Thurston, "Care in Depth," *American Journal of Nursing* 64, no. 2 (February 1964): 124.

85. Melvin J. Krant, "Letter to the Editor: 'Helping Patients Die Well,'" *New England Journal of Medicine* 280, no. 4 (January 23, 1969): 222; see also Alan Sheldon, Carol Pierson Ryser, and Melvin J. Krant, "An Integrated Family Orientated Cancer Care Program: The Report of a Pilot Project in the Socio-emotional Management of Chronic Disease," *Journal of Chronic Diseases* 22, no. 11 (April 1970): 743–55.

Chapter 2. Doctor and Nurse

The names of all patients and family members are pseudonyms. In addition, I have altered information about those individuals that could be used to identify them.

1. Julie Fairman and Joan Lynaugh, *Critical Care Nursing: A History* (Philadelphia: University of Pennsylvania Press, 1998); Arlene W. Keeling, *Nursing and the Privilege of Prescription, 1893–2000* (Columbus: Ohio State University Press, 2007).

2. Florence Wald, "Emerging Nursing Practice." *American Journal of Public Health* 56, no. 8 (1966): 1253–60.

3. "Draft of Restatement," September 25, 1969, File 12.

4. See Dan A. Oren, *Joining the Club: A History of Jews and Yale* (New Haven: Yale University Press, 1985).

5. Ira S. Goldenberg, "Preterminal Phase of Life," December 1968, File 3.

6. "Tompkins V Total Patient Care Conference," March 9, 1971, File 77.

7. Keeling, *Nursing and the Privilege of Prescription*, 118.

8. Florence S. Wald and Robert C. Leonard, "Towards Development of Nursing Practice Theory," *Nursing Research* 13, no. 4 (Fall 1964): 311.

9. Katherine Klaus, personal interview, North Haven, Connecticut, November 28, 2016.

10. "Research Conference," September 25, 1969, File 12.

11. "Data Analysis," November 4, 1970, File 65.

12. "Research Conference," September 25, 1969, File 12.

13. January 12, 1970, File 71.

14. "Dana Office," February 4, 1970, File 21.

15. "Dr. G's office," October 20, 1969, File 13.

16. Laura L. Simms, "The Hospital Staff Nurse Positions as Viewed by Baccalaureate Graduates in Nursing" (PhD diss., Teachers College, Columbia University, New York, 1963), quoted in Wald, "Emerging Nursing Practice," 1257.

17. "Dr. G's office," October 20, 1969, Filc 13.

18. "Conference with Mrs. Spina, Dana II," October 31, 1969, File 14.

19. "Dome," February 4, 1970, File 21.

20. Monica Mills, "Interview with Florence Wald," Oral History Archive, Connecticut Women's Hall of Fame, June 10, 2003.

21. "Conversation with Fr. Canny," January 26, 1970, File 72.

22. "Soundview Conv. Hosp.," October 6, 1970, File 63.

23. "Long Range Planning," September 2, 1970, File 59.

24. "Dana II," February 4, 1970, File 21.

25. "Conversation with KK, FW, and Dr. G," November 4, 1970, File 65.

26. "FW," July 29, 1970, File 53.

27. "Pt's Home," February 15, 1970, Filc 74.

28. Geritol is the trademarked name for a variety of dietary supplements believed to relieve fatigue. An investigation conducted by the Federal Trade Commission between 1959 and 1965 concluded that the mixture was ineffective for all but a small minority of people. See "Geritol's Bitter Pill," *Time*, February 5, 1973.

29. "Weekly Conference in Dome," March 18, 1969, File 31.

30. Ira S. Goldenberg, "Carcinoma of the Female Breast: Current Thoughts," *Connecticut Medicine* 30, no. 6 (June 1966): 396.

31. "Winchester 1," July 29, 1970, File 53.

32. "Winchester 1."

33. "Soundview Continuing Care," October 6, 1970, File 62.

34. "Winchester 1," July 28, 1970, File F53.

35. Nicholas A. Christakis, *Death Foretold: Prophecy and Prognosis in Medical Care* (Chicago, University of Chicago Press, 1999).

36. "Beaumont Room," February 4, 1969, File 3.

37. Barron H. Lerner, *The Good Doctor: A Father, a Son, and the Evolution of Medical Ethics* (Boston: Beacon Press, 2014), 62.

38. "Conference Goldenberg, Klaus, Wald," November 4, 1970, File 65.

39. "Conference Goldenberg, Klaus, Wald."

40. Larry Hirschhorn, "Alternative Services and the Crisis of the Professions," in *Co-ops, Communes, and Collectives*, ed. John Case and Rosemary C. R. Taylor (New York: Panthcon, 1979), 170.

41. "In Car," December 8, 1970, File 67.

42. Christakis, *Death Foretold*.

43. "Winchester 1," July 30, File 53.

44. Raymond S. Duff and August B. Hollingshead, *Sickness and Society* (New York: Harper and Row, 1968), 310.

45. Barney G. Glaser and Anselm L. Strauss, *Awareness of Dying* (New Brunswick: Aldine Transaction, 1965), 186.

46. Christakis, *Death Foretold*; Elizabeth B. Lamont and Nicholas A. Christakis, "Prognostic Disclosure to Patients with Cancer near the End of Life," *Annals of Internal Medicine* 134, no. 12 (June 19, 2001): 1096–1105; Thomas J. Smith et al., "A Pilot Trial of Decision Aids to Give Truthful Prognostic and Treatment Information to Chemotherapy Patients with Advanced Cancer," *Supportive Oncology* 9, no. 2 (March/April 2011): 79–84; Paula Span, "What Doctors Know about How Bad It Is, and Won't Say," *New York Times*, July 7, 2016.

47. "Dana II Clinic," October 23, 1969, File 13.

48. "Dana II Clinic," September 3, 1970, File 59.

49. "Dana II Clinic," September 8, 1970, File 59.

50. "Methodology Conference," February 17, 1971, File 75.

51. "Dana II Clinic," November 6, 1970, File 66.

52. "Dana II Clinic," December 4, 1970, File 67.

53. "Dana II Clinic," December 21, 1970, File 69.

54. "Home Visit," January 20, 1971, File 72.

55. "Tompkins," February 3, 1971, File 73.

56. "Tompkins," February 4, 1971, File 73.

57. "Conference," September 23, 1970, File 61.

58. July 13, 1971, File 83.

59. "Methodology Conference," February 17, 1971, File 75.

60. "Conference," September 2, 1970, File 59.

61. "Ira S. Goldenberg, Curriculum Vitae," File 2.

62. "Verbatim Report," January 8, 1970, File 18.

63. "Conversation between Diers, Wald, and Andersen," January 9, 1970, File 19.

64. "Dana II," December 1, 1969, File 16.

65. "Dana II."

66. Craig Henderson and George P. Canelios, "Cancer of the Breast—The Past Decade," *New England Journal of Medicine* 302 (1980): 17–30; Free Dictionary Medical Dictionary, s.v. "Hypophysectomy," accessed June 14, 2015, http://medical-dictionary.thefreedictionary.com/hypophysectomy. I wish to thank Barron Lerner for answering my questions about the procedure.

67. Linda Lear, *Rachel Carson, Witness for Nature* (New York: Henry Holt, 1997), 478–83.

68. Collins, W. F., "Hypophysectomy: Historical and Personal Perspective," *Clinical Neurosurgery* 21 (1974): 68–78; "William F. Collins, Jr., MD.," Society of Neurological Surgeons, accessed June 7, 2015, http://www .societyns.org/society/bio.aspx?MemberID.

69. "Dictation," December 24, 1969, File 17.

70. See Ruth R. Fader and Tom L. Beauchamp, *A History and Theory of Informed Consent* (New York: Oxford University Press, 1986); David J. Rothman, *Strangers at the Bedside* (New Brunswick: Transaction, 1991).

71. Louis W. Conway and William F. Collins, "Results of Trans-Sphenoidal Cryohypophysectomy for Carcinoma of the Breast," *New England Journal of Medicine* 281, no. 1 (July 3, 1969): 1.

72. Goldenberg, "Carcinoma," 396.

73. "Dictation," December 24, 1969, File 17.

74. Conway and Collins, "Results."

75. "Dictation," December 24, 1969, File 17.

76. "Dictation"; "TW1," December 24, 1969, File 17; "T3," December 24, 1969, File 17.

77. "T3."

78. Nancy Tomes, *Remaking the American Patient: How Madison Avenue and Modern Medicine Turned Patients into Consumers* (Chapel Hill: University of North Carolina, 2016), 182–83. For complaints about doctors performing unnecessary procedures to buy their wives fur coats, see Jim Gauger, *The Memo Book* (Bloomington: Xlibris, 2010), 431; Eleanor McBean, *The Poisoned Needle* (CreateSpace Independent Publishing Platform, 2003), 190.

79. "T3," December 24, 1969, File 17.

80. "Interdisciplinary Study of the Care of Dying Patients and Their Families," January 8, 1970, File 18.

81. "Interdisciplinary Study of the Care of Dying Patients and Their Families."

82. "Verbatim Conversation between Mrs. Wald and Dr. Goldenberg," January 16, 1970, File 19.

83. "Interdisciplinary Study of the Care of Dying Patients and Their Families," January 8, 1970, File 18.

84. "Interdisciplinary Study of the Care of Dying Patients and Their Families."

85. "Verbatim Proceedings," February 12, 1970, File 22.

86. "Weekly Conference in Dome," March 18, 1970, File 31.

87. "Verbatim Proceedings," March 19, 1970, File 32.

88. "Dana II," February 4, 1970, File 21; "Verbatim Proceedings," February 12, 1970, File 22.

89. Conway and Collins, "Results," 1.

90. "Interdisciplinary Study of the Care of Dying Patients and Their Families," January 8, 1970, File 18; "Conversation between Diers, Wald, and Andersen," February 4, 1970, File 21.

91. "Dana II," February 4, 1970, File 21; Patient #2, February 12, 1970, File 23.

92. See Paul S. Appelbaum and Charles W. Lidz, "The Therapeutic Misconception," in *Oxford Textbook of Clinical Research Ethics* (New York: Oxford University Press, 2008), 633–44.

93. "Wald and Fabric," February 19, 1970, File 25.

94. "Wald and Fabric."

95. "Verbatim Report," February 26, 1970, File 27.

96. "Bruce Fabric," February 20, 1970, File 26.

97. "Goldenberg and Wald," February 19, 1970, File 25.

98. "Verbatim Report," February 26, 1970, File 27.

99. John C. VanGilder and Ira S. Goldenberg, "Hypophysectomy in Metastatic Breast Cancer," *JAMA Surgery*, 110 (March 1975): 295.

100. "Interview with Ira Goldenberg," March 3, 1970, File 28.

101. "Pt's. Home, Hunter Radiation Therapy," April 16, 1970, File 34.

Chapter 3. Caring across Cultures

I refer to people by their first names when other people in the family have the same last name.

1. "Fitkin 1," March 25, 1969, Folder 7.
2. See Barney G. Glaser and Anselm L. Strauss, *Time for Dying* (New Brunswick: Transaction, 2007), 204–5; Alan M. Kraut, *Silent Travelers: Germs, Genes, and the "Immigrant Menace"* (New York: Basic Books, 1994).
3. "Transcription of Conversation," n.d., File 3.
4. Robert A. Orsi, *The Madonna of 115th Street*, 3rd ed. (New Haven: Yale University Press, 2002); Anthony V. Riccio, *The Italian American Experience in New Haven: Images and Oral Histories* (Albany: State University of New York Press, 2002).
5. "Tape 13," March 10, 1969, File 4.
6. Emily K. Abel, *The Inevitable Hour: A History of Caring for Dying Patients in America* (Baltimore: Johns Hopkins University Press, 2013), 46–47.
7. George Weisz, *Chronic Disease in the Twentieth Century, A History* (Baltimore: Johns Hopkins University Press, 2014), 137.
8. Franz Goldmann, "Patients in Chronic Disease Hospitals: A Profile," *American Journal of Public Health* 52, no. 4 (1962): 646–55.
9. Sheila M. Rothman, "Review of George Weisz, *Chronic Disease in the Twentieth Century,*" *American Historical Review* (December 2015): 1866–67.
10. "Notes Dictated on Ward H5," n.d., File 3.
11. Abel, *Inevitable Hour*.
12. "Nurses Sitting Room," February 11, 1969, File 4.
13. Barney G. Glaser and Anselm L. Strauss, *Awareness of Dying*, 3rd reprint (New Brunswick: Aldine Transaction, 2007), 136.
14. "Conference with Schenk, Blood and Wald," February 11, 1969, File 5.
15. "Sitting Room," February 11, 1969, File 4.
16. "Office of Supervisor of Norwalk VNA," February 13, 1969, File 4.
17. "Maestro," n.d., File 4.
18. Orsi, *Madonna*.

19. February 17, file 5; "Olivia Vlahos and FSW," March 10, 1969, File 6.

20. "Conference," February 27, 1969, File 5.

21. Barney G. Glaser and Anselm L. Strauss, "The Social Loss of Dying Patients," *American Journal of Nursing* 64, no. 6 (June 1964): 121.

22. "Conference," February 27, 1969, File 5; "Olivia Vlahos and FSW," March 10, 1969, File 6.

23. "Conference."

24. "Olivia Vlahos and FSW," March 10, 1969, File 6.

25. "Conference," February 27, 1969, File 5.

26. Dan A. Oren, *Joining the Club: A History of Jews and Yale* (New Haven: Yale University Press, 1985), 364–65.

27. "Conference," February 27, 1969, File 5.

28. "Conference."

29. "Olivia Vlahos and FSW," March 10, 1969, File 6.

30. "Conference," February 27, 1969, File 5.

31. "Conference."

32. "Olivia Vlahos and FSW," March 10, 1969, File 6.

33. "Summary of Past Four Weeks," March 28, 1969, File 6.

34. "Office of Chaplain E. Dobihal," March 12, 1969, File 6.

35. "Fitkin I," March 18, 1969, File 6.

36. "Office of Chaplain E. Dobihal," March 12, 1969, File 6.

37. "Olivia Vlahos and FSW," March 10, 1969, File 6.

38. "Beaumont Room," March 28, 1969, File 7.

39. "Beaumont Room"; see Riccio, *Italian American Experience*, 193.

40. Abel, *Inevitable Hour*.

41. "Wald House," March 28, 1969, File 8.

42. "FII, March 14, 1969," File 7.

43. "Wald Home," April 28, 1969, File 8.

44. "Telephone Call," July 7, 1969, File 8.

45. "Notes of August 6," August 6, 1969, File 8.

46. Joel Wald, telephone interview, January 20, 2017.

47. "Home of patient's daughter, office of the state welfare worker in Norwalk," October 9, 1969, File 13.

48. "Conversation with Mrs. Rossi," November 25, 1969, File 15.

49. "Home of the Patient," March 1, 1970, file 28.

Chapter 4. Hope, Blame, and Acceptance

1. Barron H. Lerner, *The Breast Cancer Wars: Hope, Fear, and the Pursuit of a Cure in Twentieth-Century America* (New York: Oxford University Press, 2001), 15–78.

2. Frederick L. Greene, "Remembering Ira," *General Surgery News* 35, no. 12 (December 2008).

3. Lerner, *Breast Cancer Wars*, 15–240; James S. Olson, *Bathsheba's Breast: Women, Cancer, and History* (Baltimore: Johns Hopkins University Press, 2002), 67, 89.

4. Terese Lasser, "I Had Breast Cancer," *Coronet* (April 1954): 109.

5. Lerner, *Breast Cancer Wars*, 191–93.

6. Kirsten E. Gardner, *Early Detection: Women, Cancer, and Awareness Campaigns in the Twentieth-Century United States* (Chapel Hill, University of North Carolina Press, 2006), 147–54.

7. Gardner, *Early Detection*, 106.

8. Keith Wailoo, *How Cancer Crossed the Color Line* (New York: Oxford University Press, 2011), 72–74.

9. Gardner, *Early Detection*, 146.

10. December 1, 1969, File 16.

11. "Research Conference, Steiner Room," February 12, 1970, File 22.

12. "Verbatim Proceedings," February 12, 1970, File 22.

13. "Verbatim Proceedings," April 1, 1970, File 33.

14. "Dr. G's Office," March 20, 1970, File 33.

15. "Wald and Goldenberg in Goldenberg's Office," February 19, 1969, File 25.

16. "Following the Research Conference in the Beaumont Room," December 4, 1969, File 16.

17. "Dana II," February 18, 1970, File 23.

18. "Patient's Home," February 27, 1970, File 28.

19. "Patient's Home."

20. March 13, 1970, File 30.

21. "Dana II," February 18, 1970, File 23.

22. "Dome Office," March 3, 1970, Folder 29.

23. "Verbatim Proceedings," February 26, 1970, File 27.

24. "Dome Office," March 19, 1970, File 29.

25. "Verbatim Proceedings," March 19, 1970, File 32.

26. "Reconstruction from Memory," June 4, 1970, File 35.

27. "Dictation," March 16, 1970, File 30.

28. "Verbatim Proceedings," May 13, 1970, File 37.

29. Hildegard E. Peplau, *Interpersonal Relations in Nursing: A Conceptual Frame of Reference for Psychodynamic Nursing* (New York: Springer, 1991), 79.

30. "Research Record," April 20, 1970, File 35.

31. "Pt's Home, Woodbridge Country Club," April 16, 1970, File 34.

32. "Conference," October 6, 1970, File 62.

33. "WIII," June 4, 1970, File 35.

34. "WIII," April 27, 1970, File 35.

35. Bruce C. Vladeck, *Unloving Care: The Nursing Home Tragedy* (New York: Basic Books, 1980), 104–5.

36. Sheila B Amdur and Marilyn Beach, "Mrs. Lucia Hawkins, L. P. N.," n.d., File 9.

37. "W3," April 28, 1970, File 36.

38. "Winchester III Staff Conference," January 14, 1970, File 71.

39. Barbara Melosh, *"The Physician's Hand": Work, Conflict, and Culture in American Nursing* (Philadelphia: Temple University Press, 1982).

40. Arthur W. Frank, *At the Will of the Body* (Boston: Houghton Mifflin, 1991), 79.

41. "Hawkins Home," May 8, 1970, File 37.

42. "Mrs. Hawkins home," May 11, 1970, File 37.

43. "Office and Home," May 14, 1970, File 38.

44. "Verbatim Proceedings," May 13, 1970, File 38.

45. Elisabeth Kübler-Ross, *On Death and Dying* (New York: Scribner, 1969), 124.

46. "Driving on Way to Lake Waramaug," May 15, 16, 18, 1970, File 38.

47. "Thumbnail Sketch," May 8, 1970, File 36.

48. "Reconstruction from Memory," May 8–11, 1970, File 36.

49. "WIII," April 27, 1970, File 35.

50. "Driving on Way to Lake Waramaug," May 15, 16, 18, 1970, File 38.

51. "Conversation between K. Klaus and F. Wald in Brady Classroom," April 29, 1970, File 35.

52. "Conversation between K. Klaus and F. Wald in Brady Classroom."

53. "W3," May 31, 1970, File 40.

54. "Patient's Home," May 31, 1970, File 40.

55. "Telephone Call to Pt's Sister," June 12, 1970, File 44.

56. "Dictation," July 8, 1970, File 47.

57. "Conference," October 6, 1970, File 63.

58. Frank, *At the Will of the Body*.

Chapter 5. Making Sense of the Findings

1. "Conference between FW and DD," April 7, 1971, File 79.

2. Florence Wald, "In Search of the Spiritual Component of Hospice Care," in *In Quest of the Spiritual Component of Care for the Terminally Ill: Proceedings of a Colloquium, May 3–4, 1986, Yale University School of Nursing*, ed. Florence Wald (New Haven: 1986), 31. Copyright Florence Wald.

3. Mary Jo Maynes, Jennifer L. Pierce, and Barbara Laslett, *Telling Stories: The Uses of Personal Narratives in the Social Sciences and History* (Ithaca: Cornell University Press, 2008).

4. "M. French's Office," August 5, 1970, File 54.

5. "Methodology Conference," April 24, 1970, File 79.

6. Emily K. Abel, *The Inevitable Hour: A History of Caring for Dying Patients in America* (Baltimore: Johns Hopkins Press, 2013).

7. "Conference," September 11, 1969, File 11.

8. "Staff Conference with Mrs. Weber and Various Nurses," January 14, 1971, File 71.

9. "Tompkins 4," July 29, 1969, File 10.

10. Bruce C. Vladeck, *Unloving Care: The Nursing Home Tragedy* (New York: Basic Books, 1980).

11. "Data Analysis," November 4, 1970, File 65.

12. "Dana II," May 11, 1970, File 37.

13. Philippe Ariès, *The Hour of Our Death* (New York: Vintage Books, 1981), 568–70.

14. "Conference," November 13, 1969, File 14.

15. "Pt's Apartment," June 16, 1970, File 44.

16. "To Honor All Life: A National Demonstration Center to Protect the Rights of the Terminally Ill, the Case for Support of Hospice, Inc.," File 23, pp. 5, 16.

17. "To Honor All Life," pp. 1, 5.

18. Emily K. Abel, *Living in Death's Shadow: Family Experiences of Terminal Illness and Irreplaceable Loss* (Baltimore: Johns Hopkins University Press, 2017), 126–27.

19. Barney G. Glaser and Anselm L. Strauss, *Time for Dying* (New Brunswick: Aldine Transaction, 1998), 14.

20. "W3," May 4, 1970, File 36.

21. "Patient Data Conf.," March 3, 1971, File 76.

22. "Data Analysis," June 10, 1970, File 43.

23. "Dana II Clinic," October 5, 1970, File 62.

24. "Conversation between Klaus, Wald, and Phipps," December 11, 1970, File 68.

25. "Dana Clinic," February 19, 1971, File 75.

26. Ann Bradshaw, "The Spiritual Dimension of Hospice: The Secularization of an Ideal," *Social Science and Medicine* 43, no. 3 (1996): 409–19; David Clark, "Religion, Medicine, and Community in the Early Origins of St. Christopher's Hospice," *Journal of Palliative Medicine* 4, no. 3 (2001): 353–60.

27. "Conference," September 1, 1970, File 54.

28. Shari Wald Vogler, phone interview, December 20, 2016.

29. "Notes from Meeting with Cicely Saunders," January 5, 1971, File 68.

30. "Dana Clinic," June 7, 1971, File 82.

31. "Cove Manor," August 9, 1971, File 84.

32. "Cove Manor," August 16, 1971, File 84.

33. "Maestro," n.d., File 4.

34. "Staff Conference," January 13, 1971, File 27.

35. "Verbatim Proceedings," April 1, 1970, File 33.

36. "WWI," August 24, 1979, File 56.

37. "Verbatim Transcript of Visit to Staff of T2," August 28, 1970, File 57.

38. Joan Craven and Florence S. Wald, "Hospice Care for Dying Patients," *American Journal of Nursing* 75, no. 10 (Oct. 1975): 1821.

39. "T-5," November 17, 1969, File 15.

40. "WIII," February 13, 1970, File 23.

41. "Team Conference on WI," September 1, 1970, File 58.

42. "Staff Conference with Mrs. Weber and Group of Nurses," January 14, 1971, File 71.

43. "Verbatim Proceedings," February 27, 1970, File 27.

44. Julian Barnes, *Something to Declare*, quoted in Pamela Druckerman, "France, Paradise Lost," *New York Times*, November 3, 2015.

Conclusion

1. "In Memoriam: YSN Dean Florence Wald, Founder of Hospice Care in the U.S.," *Yale News*, November 21, 2008, http://news.yale.edu/2008/11/21/memoriam-ysn-dean-florence-wald-founder-hospice-care.

2. Edward F. Dobihal and Charles William Stewart, *When a Friend Is Dying: A Guide to Caring for the Terminally Ill and Bereaved* (Nashville: Abingdon Press, 1984).

3. "The Rev. Edward Dobihal," *Making an Impact: Supporting the Mission of Yale–New Haven Hospital* (Summer 2009), 14–15.

4. Ira S. Goldenberg, "Hospice: To Humanize Dying," *Bulletin of the American College of Surgeons* 64, no. 2 (April 1979): 9.

5. Frederick L. Greene, "Remembering Ira," *General Surgery News* 35, no. 12 (December 2008).

6. David S. Fischer, *The Clinical Cancer Program at Yale* (New Haven: Yale Printing and Publishing Services, 2012), 43.

7. Nancy Polk, "A Much-Loved New Haven Doctor Retires," *New York Times*, July 25, 1993.

8. Katherine Klaus, personal interview, North Haven, Connecticut, October 29, 2016.

9. Carole Bass, "Donna Diers, Living Legend of Nursing, Dies," *Yale Alumni Magazine*, February 27, 2013; Sharon Eck Birmingham and Suzanne M. Boyle, "A Legacy of Data Use by Donna Diers," *Nursing Economics* 31, no. 3 (May/June 2013): 144; Diana J. Mason, "In Memoriam: Donna Diers," *American Journal of Nursing* 113, no. 4 (April 2013): 19; Colleen Shaddox, "A Former Dean, But Never a Former Nurse," *Yale Alumni Magazine*, May/June 2013.

10. See, for example, Robert W. Buckingham, *The Complete Hospice Guide* (New York: Harper and Row, 1983); Parker Rossman, *Hospice: Creating*

New Models for the Terminally Ill (New York: Fawcett Columbine, 1977); and Sandol Stoddard, *The Hospice Movement: A Better Way of Caring for the Dying* (New York: Vintage, 1978).

11. Buckingham, *Hospice Guide*, 28–29.

12. Rossman, *Hospice*, 122.

13. Buckingham, *Hospice Guide*, 29.

14. Florence Wald, "Hospice Care in the United States," in *Facing Death*, ed. Howard M. Spiro, Mary G. McCrea Curnen, and Lee Palmer Wandel (New Haven: Yale University Press, 1996), 86.

15. Rossman, *Hospice*, 30.

16. Using a discourse analysis, Camilla Zimmermann found that acceptance of death remains a central concept in various forms of palliative care. See Camilla Zimmermann, "Acceptance of Dying: A Discourse Analysis of Palliative Care Literature," *Social Science and Medicine* 75 (2012): 217–24.

17. Feather Ann Davis, "Medicare Hospice Benefit: Early Program Experiences," *Health Care Financing Review* 9, no. 4 (Summer 1988): 99; MedPac Commission, "Chapter 11," *Hospice Services*, 285, accessed Oct. 10, 2015, http://www.medpac.gov/documents/MedPac_.

18. National Hospice and Palliative Care Organization, *NHPCO's Facts and Figures: Hospice Care in America* (Alexandria: National Hospice and Palliative Care Organization, 2013), 4; MedPac, "Chapter 11."

19. Joan Teno, quoted in Peter Whoriskey and Dan Keating, "Rising Rates of Hospice Discharge in U.S. Raise Questions about Quality of Care," *Washington Post*, August 6, 2014.

Acknowledgments

I wish to thank Cynthia Connolly, Katherine Klaus, Shari Vogler, and Joel Wald for sharing their memories of Florence Wald; Rick Abel, Carla Bittel, Janet Brodie, Sharla Fett, Alice Wexler, for reading various chapters; Patricia D'Antonio for reviewing the manuscript for Rutgers University Press; and Barron H. Lerner for providing critical medical information.

I also am grateful to Archives and Manuscripts, Yale University Library, New Haven, for permission to quote from the Florence and Henry Wald Papers (MS 1659).

Index

Page numbers in *italics* refer to figures.

prejudice: ethnic, 53, 58, 66–67, 90; gender, 30, 95–96; racial, 61, 90; religious, 18, 28; socioeconomic, 59–60, 63, 80, 91, 94

prolongation of life, 21, 23, 67, 92. *See also* health care: curative

psychoanalysis, 4, 13, 17, 91

quality of life, 23, 116
Quint, Jeanne C., 22, 25, 89

radiation, 37–38, 43, 116
Ramsey, Paul, 23
Reach to Recovery, 69–70, 71–72
Reader's Digest, 23
Redlich, Frederick C., 14
religion, 11, 58–59, 83, 101–2; and death, 23. *See also* Catholicism; clergy; Judaism; prejudice: religious
rooming in, 17
Rossi, Allegra, 58, 60, 63–64, 65–66, 106
Rossi, Nunzio, 52–67, 92; death, 65; family conflicts, 53–54, 58, 60–61, 63–64, 67, 104, 112–13; finances, 61, 102; home care, 58, 60–62, 94–95; hospitalization, 52, 62; IV difficulties, 56, 58, 59, 62
Rossi, Robert, 53–55, 57–58, 64–65, 66, 67, 112
Rossman, Parker, 112
"Routinization of Hospice, The," 1–2
Rutgers University School of Nursing, 13
Rynearson, Edward H., 23

Saint Christopher's in the Field, 2, 102
Saint Raphael's Hospital, 54
Saunders, Cicely, 2, 10, 15–16, 102
Schorske, Carl E., 30
Shenk, Ian M., 56–59
Sickness and Society, 14–15
social change movements, 19–20
Social Class and Mental Illness: A Community Study, 14
Social Security Act, 56
sociologists, 22
Spock, Benjamin, 17, 20

stages of grief, 6–7, 21, 83; acceptance, 7, 83, 99–100, 102, 114–15; denial, 72, 79; depression, 81; questioning of, 99, 115
Steinberg (doctor), 65
Strange, John, 96, 97
Strauss, Anselm L., 22, 40, 89
Sudnow, David, 22

theologians, 23
therapeutic misconception, 49
Time for Dying, 22

United Kingdom, 2, 102
U.S. Public Health Service, 3

Vietnam War, 20
Visiting Nurse Association, 58
Vladeck, Bruce C., 80–81
Vogler, Shari Wald, 11, 14, 78

Wald, Florence Schorske, *12*; attitude toward death, 71; background, 10–11; and Ruth Cohen, 43–51; data presentation, 89–90, 104, 108; on doctor-nurse relationship, 30; education, 11; emotional transference, 4, 106–7; empathy, 80; family relationships, 3, 4, 89; and Ira Goldenberg, 28, 31–34, 47–48, 51, 114; and Alice Hirsch, 74, 76, 85–86, 88, 96–97, 112; honesty, 43, 72, 113; and Hospice Inc., 109; hospice movement foundation, 1; idealization of cases, 9, 104–5; and Mrs. Klein, 84–85; later career, 109; management style, 15, 109; medical competency, 92; medical staff relationships, 51, 62–63, 67, 93–94; overinvolvement, 4, 59, 62–63, 78, 86; patient relationships, 64, 89; personal traits, 4; prejudices, 55, 90–91; and religion, 11, 101–2; and Allegra Rossi, 60, 63, 65–66, 67; and Nunzio Rossi, 52–54, 55, 58–59, 61; and Rossi family, 53–54, 65–66, 67; and social change movements, 20; sparing family distress, 96, 113; and "stages of grief" theory, 7, 83,

About the Author

EMILY K. ABEL is professor emerita at the Fielding-UCLA School of Public Health. She has published many books on the history of medicine and public health, including *Hearts of Wisdom: American Women Caring for Kin, 1850–1940*; *The Inevitable Hour: A History of Caring for Dying Patients in America*; and *Living in Death's Shadow: Family Experiences of Terminal Care and Irreplaceable Loss*.

Available titles in the Critical Issues in Health and Medicine series:

James A. Schafer Jr., *The Business of Private Medical Practice: Doctors, Specialization, and Urban Change in Philadelphia, 1900–1940*

David G. Schuster, *Neurasthenic Nation: America's Search for Health, Happiness, and Comfort, 1869–1920*

Karen Seccombe and Kim A. Hoffman, *Just Don't Get Sick: Access to Health Care in the Aftermath of Welfare Reform*

Leo B. Slater, *War and Disease: Biomedical Research on Malaria in the Twentieth Century*

Dena T. Smith, *Medicine over Mind: Mental Health Practice in the Biomedical Era*

Matthew Smith, *An Alternative History of Hyperactivity: Food Additives and the Feingold Diet*

Paige Hall Smith, Bernice L. Hausman, and Miriam Labbok, *Beyond Health, Beyond Choice: Breastfeeding Constraints and Realities*

Susan L. Smith, *Toxic Exposures: Mustard Gas and the Health Consequences of World War II in the United States*

Rosemary A. Stevens, Charles E. Rosenberg, and Lawton R. Burns, eds., *History and Health Policy in the United States: Putting the Past Back In*

Barbra Mann Wall, *American Catholic Hospitals: A Century of Changing Markets and Missions*

Frances Ward, *The Door of Last Resort: Memoirs of a Nurse Practitioner*

Shannon Withycombe, *Lost: Miscarriage in Nineteenth-Century America*

Printed and bound by CPI Group (UK) Ltd, Croydon, CR0 4YY

27/10/2024

14580231-0001